Cardiac Sarcoidosis

Andrew M. Freeman • Howard D. Weinberger
Editors

Cardiac Sarcoidosis

Key Concepts in Pathogenesis, Disease
Management, and Interesting Cases

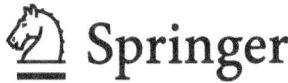 Springer

Editors
Andrew M. Freeman
Department of Medicine
Division of Cardiology
National Jewish Health
Denver, CO
USA

Howard D. Weinberger
Department of Medicine
Division of Cardiology
National Jewish Health
Denver, CO
USA

ISBN 978-3-319-35679-2   ISBN 978-3-319-14624-9 (eBook)
DOI 10.1007/978-3-319-14624-9

Springer Cham Heidelberg New York Dordrecht London
© Springer International Publishing Switzerland 2015
Softcover re-print of the Hardcover 1st edition 2015
This work is subject to copyright. All rights are reserved by the Publisher, whether the whole or part of the material is concerned, specifically the rights of translation, reprinting, reuse of illustrations, recitation, broadcasting, reproduction on microfilms or in any other physical way, and transmission or information storage and retrieval, electronic adaptation, computer software, or by similar or dissimilar methodology now known or hereafter developed.
The use of general descriptive names, registered names, trademarks, service marks, etc. in this publication does not imply, even in the absence of a specific statement, that such names are exempt from the relevant protective laws and regulations and therefore free for general use.
The publisher, the authors and the editors are safe to assume that the advice and information in this book are believed to be true and accurate at the date of publication. Neither the publisher nor the authors or the editors give a warranty, express or implied, with respect to the material contained herein or for any errors or omissions that may have been made.

Printed on acid-free paper

Springer is part of Springer Science+Business Media (www.springer.com)

Preface

Sarcoidosis remains an elusive diagnosis even in this day and age with fantastic technology available in nearly any sizeable city. Further, once diagnosed, the disease can be progressive and disabling or remain quiescent for years. It can affect any organ, but of course, one of the greatest concerns is cardiac involvement which can lead to sudden death, arrhythmia, and heart failure, in addition to a great many other complications.

This handbook is meant to serve as a clinician's field guide to diagnosing, managing, and treating cardiac sarcoidosis. Much of the epidemiology, pathophysiology, and treatments are reviewed with a strong clinical angle to all discussions in an effort to provide high yield and immediately implementable concepts at the bedside. You will find clear commentary on virtually any situation to be encountered in this disease process and clear direction on how to proceed in diagnosing and managing the disease. The major caveat is that there is still no gold standard in diagnosing the disease, and even worse, no strong consensus on treatment options. Despite this, our authors have worked hard to present evidence-based and balanced approaches, and in areas with little to no evidence, we have clearly attempted to provide best practice.

You will notice that each chapter ends with "Pearls of Wisdom." This is our attempt to provide some of the deep wisdom in the text of the chapter in a very high yield and manageable chunk for those who might be pressed for time. A thorough read of each chapter should provide the depth of knowledge that will then also be reinforced by these Pearls. The book ends with case examples to guide clinicians through real-world case scenarios with actual management situations described in detail. Our hope is to provide a beacon of light through the sometimes murky waters of cardiac sarcoidosis.

While all sections of this guide are equally strong, some notable sections include an in-depth discussion on the possibilities for pathogenesis, and a clear focus on multi-modality imaging, and management with immunosuppression. The research as of late in this field has clouded the understanding of where this disease emanates from, but the section on pathophysiology should give the reader some understanding of the very heterogeneous environment that may result in the disease state. As mentioned, there is no clear cut algorithm for diagnosing the disease, which, in the current era is largely dependent on advanced imaging diagnostics. The imaging sections, and notably the multi-modality section, will serve to anchor the clinician in making good decisions in this realm of many possible approaches. While little evidence supports various immunosuppression regimens, the sections on treatment will serve to provide perspective in this arena where little guidance exists.

In sum, we hope you will find this guide an easy-to-access, in-depth, and well-indexed guide for the latest in diagnosis and treatment of this complicated and challenging disease.

Denver, CO, USA   Andrew M. Freeman, MD, FACC, FACP

Introduction: Overview of Cardiac Sarcoidosis

Sarcoidosis is a multi-system granulomatous disease characterized by non-caseating granulomas. The etiology for this granulomatous response is unknown. Sarcoidosis primarily affects the lungs, but extra-pulmonary sarcoidosis can affect any organ system. Cardiac sarcoidosis is the most feared, as the repercussions can be severe, life threatening and can occur without warning. The first described case of cardiac sarcoidosis was reported by Bernstein in 1929, who described sarcoidosis granulomas in the pericardium [1].

There are several features of cardiac involvement of sarcoidosis which are different from almost all other organs involved by sarcoidosis. Two of the most common complications of cardiac sarcoidosis may occur suddenly, without warning in an otherwise normal appearing heart, and may be fatal on the initial presentation. These include interference or disruption of the electrical conduction system including complete heart block, AV block or bundle branch blocks and ventricular arrhythmias and sudden cardiac death. These potentially life threatening complications may occur as a result of scarring and the healing process after acute inflammation and "active disease" has subsided. In addition, as both sarcoidosis disease activity and response to therapy may be variable over time, it is nearly impossible to rule out the potential risk for cardiac sarcoidosis and its serious or life threatening complications after a single negative evaluation.

The true incidence of cardiac involvement is difficult to determine due to the lack of a highly sensitive and specific "gold standard" test, and the apparent differences from country to country. For example, in the United States 13–25 % of deaths in patients with sarcoidosis are due to cardiac sarcoidosis while in Japan 47–85 % of deaths in patients with sarcoidosis are due to cardiac sarcoidosis. Because of these and other limitations, cardiac sarcoidosis is likely underdiagnosed. Most studies report a clinically apparent incidence of ~5 %, while autopsy studies suggest up to 70 % of patients with sarcoidosis have cardiac involvement [2]. Unfortunately, the first clinical manifestation of cardiac sarcoidosis may be sudden cardiac death or a life threatening conduction abnormality or arrhythmia. Less than half of patients with cardiac sarcoidosis found at autopsy had the diagnosis of cardiac involvement prior to death [3].

The clinician's goal is to identify, risk stratify and treat those patients with cardiac involvement before irreversible damage, or serious or life threatening complications occur. Yazaki et al. reported that instituting therapy while left ventricular systolic function was still preserved resulted in a better clinical outcome [4]. This underscores the importance of considering and looking for evidence of cardiac involvement in patients with sarcoidosis prior to the appearance of overt or serious clinical manifestations of cardiac involvement.

In this guidebook, the authors will work to take you through the various aspects of cardiac sarcoidosis – from its origins and epidemiology to presentation, diagnosis, and management. The reader will also find several clinical vignettes to aid in deepening the understanding of the ways in which cardiac sarcoidosis could present and what was done to manage its clinical manifestations.

Denver, CO, USA   Howard D. Weinberger, MD, FACC, FACP

References

1. Bernstein M, Konglemann FW, Sidlick DM. Boeck's sarcoid. Report of a case with visceral involvement. Arch Intern Med. 1929;44:721–34.
2. Bargout R, Kelly RF. Sarcoid heart disease: clinical course and treatment. Int J Cardiol. 2004;97:173–82.
3. Sekhri V, Sanal S, DeLorenzo LJ, et al. Cardiac sarcoidosis: a comprehensive review. Arch Med Sci. 2011;4:546.
4. Yazaki Y, Isobe M, Hiro M, et al. Prognostic determinants of long-term survival in Japanese patients with cardiac sarcoidosis treated with prednisone. Am J Cardiol. 2001;88:1006–10.

Contents

1. **High Yield Epidemiology** 1
   Andrew M. Freeman

2. **Pathophysiology: From Genetics to Viruses and More** 5
   Andrew M. Freeman

3. **Clinical Presentations** 11
   Howard D. Weinbeger

4. **Standard Screening for Cardiac Sarcoidosis** 15
   Andrew M. Freeman

5. **Diagnosis II: Imaging of Cardiac Sarcoidosis
   with Cardiac MRI, PET and SPECT** 25
   Joyce D. Schroeder and Brett Fenster

6. **Nuclear Imaging (SPECT and PET) in Cardiac Sarcoidosis** 39
   Ron Blankstein and Sharmila Dorbala

7. **Multimodality Imaging of Cardiac Sarcoidosis** 51
   Ron Blankstein and Edward J. Miller

8. **Invasive Procedures and Endomyocardial Biopsy** 73
   Darlene Kim and William H. Sauer

9. **Management of Arrhythmias Related to Cardiac Sarcoidosis** 81
   Matthew M. Zipse and William H. Sauer

10. **Acute Management of Cardiac Sarcoidosis** 93
    Neal K. Lakdawala and Garrick C. Stewart

11. **Immunosuppressive Management of Cardiac Sarcoidosis** 103
    Divya Patel and Nabeel Y. Hamzeh

12 **Management of Sudden Death Risk Related to Cardiac Sarcoidosis** 113
Matthew M. Zipse and William H. Sauer

13 **Sarcoidosis-Associated Pulmonary Hypertension** 125
Brett Fenster

14 **Cases in Cardiac Sarcoidosis** 135
Andrew M. Freeman, Howard D. Weinbeger, Darlene Kim, Brett Fenster, Joyce D. Schroeder, Nabeel Y. Hamzeh, William H. Sauer, Matthew M. Zipse, Divya Patel, Ron Blankstein, Sharmila Dorbala, Edward J. Miller, Neal K. Lakdawala, and Garrick C. Stewart

15 **Patient-Centered Care for Sarcoidosis** 161
Darlene Kim and Howard D. Weinberger

Sarcoidosis Resources for Patients and Caregivers 165

Index 167

Contributors

Ron Blankstein MD, FACC Non-invasive Cardiovascular Imaging Program, Department of Medicine (Cardiovascular Division) and Department of Radiology, Brigham and Women's Hospital, Harvard Medical School, Boston, MA, USA

Sharmila Dorbala MD, MPH Non-invasive Cardiovascular Imaging Program, Department of Medicine (Cardiovascular Division) and Department of Radiology, Brigham and Women's Hospital, Harvard Medical School, Boston, MA, USA

Brett Fenster MD, FACC, FACP, FASE Division of Cardiology, Department of Medicine, National Jewish Health, Denver, CO, USA

Andrew M. Freeman MD, FACC, FACP Division of Cardiology, Department of Medicine, National Jewish Health, Denver, CO, USA

Nabeel Y. Hamzeh MD Division of Environmental and Occupational Health Sciences, Department of Medicine, National Jewish Health, Denver, CO, USA

Division of Pulmonary and Critical Care Sciences, Department of Medicine, University of Colorado Hospital, Aurora, CO, USA

Darlene Kim MD, FACC Division of Cardiology, Department of Medicine, National Jewish Health, Denver, CO, USA

Neal K. Lakdawala MD Cardiovascular Medicine, Brigham and Women's Hospital, Harvard Medical School, Boston, MA, USA

Edward J. Miller MD, PhD Section of Cardiovascular Medicine, Boston University School of Medicine, Boston, MA, USA

Divya Patel DO Division of Pulmonary and Critical Care Sciences, Department of Medicine, University of Colorado Hospital, Aurora, CO, USA

William H. Sauer MD Section of Cardiac Electrophysiology, Division of Cardiology, University of Colorado Hospital, Aurora, CO, USA

Joyce D. Schroeder MD Department of Radiology, University of Colorado, Adjoint Associate Professor, Aurora, CO, USA

Garrick C. Stewart MD Cardiovascular Medicine, Brigham and Women's Hospital, Harvard Medical School, Boston, MA, USA

Howard D. Weinberger MD, FACC, FACP Division of Cardiology, Department of Medicine, National Jewish Health, Denver, CO, USA

Matthew M. Zipse MD Section of Cardiac Electrophysiology, Division of Cardiology, University of Colorado Hospital, Aurora, CO, USA

Chapter 1
High Yield Epidemiology

Andrew M. Freeman

Abstract Sarcoidosis is an intriguing, puzzling, multi-system granulomatous condition, with multiple confounding manifestations. In this section, the variations in incidence, racial and ethnic factors, and clinical presentation variations will be described in detail. Sarcoidosis most often presents in African American persons, particularly in cases described in North America, and is usually a disease of early middle age. In some parts of the world, such as Japan, the vast majority of deaths from sarcoidosis appear to be heart related, and in all likelihood, cardiac involvement is under diagnosed, owing to heterogeneous symptoms (and sometimes no symptoms at all), and the bias that results from the disease's first manifestation often being sudden cardiac death.

Sarcoidosis Epidemiology

Sarcoidosis is an intriguing, puzzling, multi-system granulomatous condition, with multiple confounding manifestations that was initially described by Dr. Caeser Boeck, a Norwegian dermatologist in 1899. He had described the lesions he saw on the skin as "epithelioid cells with large pale nuclei and also a few giant cells [1]". Prior to that, an English physician, Jonathon Hutchinson, described a patient in 1877 [2] whose hands and feet had multiple, raised, purplish cutaneous patches that which had developed the preceding 2 years. Hutchinson hypothesized these were due to gout, but then realized, later that these were likely a "form of skin disease which has hitherto escaped special recognition [3] (Fig. 1.1)."

As sarcoidosis is now more widely recognized and with increased rigor in its diagnosis, previous, older characterizations of the disease prevalence and incidence may be incorrect. Based on more recent work, the disease seems to vary widely

A.M. Freeman, MD, FACC, FACP
Division of Cardiology, Department of Medicine, National Jewish Health,
1400 Jackson St., Denver, CO 80206, USA
e-mail: freemana@njhealth.org

© Springer International Publishing Switzerland 2015
A.M. Freeman, H.D. Weinberger (eds.), *Cardiac Sarcoidosis:
Key Concepts in Pathogenesis, Disease Management, and Interesting Cases*,
DOI 10.1007/978-3-319-14624-9_1

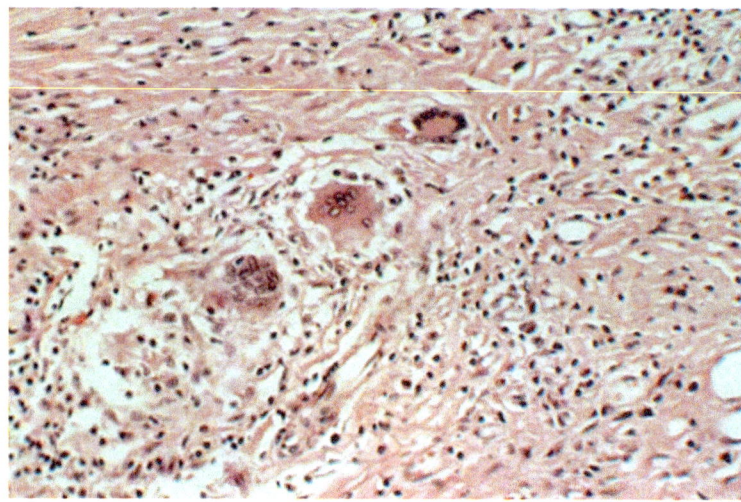

Fig. 1.1 A myocardial biopsy obtained via right heart catheterization showing giant cells consistent with sarcoidosis

throughout the world in terms of incidence. That said, it remains highly prevalent in African Americans, almost three times the annual incidence of white Americans (35.5 cases per 100,000, as compared with 10.9 per 100,000) [4]. The lifetime risk of sarcoidosis in African Americans in the United States is quoted at approximately 2.4 %, compared with a lifetime risk of 0.85 % in Caucasians [4]. It has also been well characterized in many other countries including Japan (incidence of about 2 cases per 100,000 people) [5], which has established the well-known Japanese Ministry of Health criteria for diagnosis of the disease. The highest reported incidence occurs in northern European countries and is quoted at 5–40 cases per 100,000 people [5]. Overall, the disease prevalence is estimated at 20 per 100,000 [6].

For most cases, sarcoidosis develops before middle age, usually before age 50, with peak incidence in early adulthood, ages 20–39. In Japan, the peak incidence is in the third decade, while in Americans, the incidence is later in life, usually in the fourth decade. Americans afflicted with the disease are also more likely to have chronic active disease states and are more likely to succumb to the disease [7]. Interestingly, in Scandinavia, there are two peaks for age of onset: one at 25–29 years and the other at 65–69 years of age [8]. While both sexes are affected, in all countries women seem to be more commonly affected [9]. Overall, sarcoidosis presents from 10 to 40 years of age in 70–90 % of cases. More than half of all cases are detected incidentally by radiography prior to symptoms [7].

While socioeconomic status doesn't clearly affect incidence, those of lower socioeconomic status are more likely to present later in the disease process due to the barriers of low income, lack of access to medical providers, and lower educational level. Furthermore, if adjusted for race, ethnicity, age, or gender, this higher degree of severity in this socioeconomic status persists [10].

Sarcoidosis can involve nearly any organ system, but is most often found involving the pulmonary system in more than 90 % of the cases reported. Up to

30 % of patients afflicted with the disease have extra-thoracic manifestations [7]. In addition to pulmonary involvement, it most commonly affects the skin, and eyes. Cardiac involvement is variable, but is a major cause of morbidity and mortality.

Cardiac Sarcoidosis

Clinical evidence of myocardial involvement is present in only about 5 % of patients with sarcoidosis. However, autopsy studies indicate that subclinical cardiac involvement is present in 20–30 % of cases [11]. This number may even be higher (as much as 39 % [12]) – likely because the first manifestation of cardiac sarcoidosis can be sudden cardiac death and not all patients present in time to have the diagnosis made. Myocardial involvement is common in patients with sarcoidosis who have cardiac symptoms and unusual in those without such symptoms [13].

There seem to be significant differences in how cardiac sarcoidosis presents among various countries, although comparison among studies is limited owing to differing study methodologies. In American studies, 13–25 % of deaths from sarcoidosis have been attributed to cardiac sarcoidosis while in Japan, 47–85 % of deaths from sarcoidosis have been attributed to cardiac involvement [14]. Interestingly in a smaller retrospective study from Haifa, Israel they observed just 2 of 120 patients with sarcoidosis died of cardiac involvement [15].

Cardiac sarcoidosis can often result in lethal ventricular tachyarrhythmias or conduction block, which accounts for 25–65 % of deaths [16]. Symptomatic or electrocardiographically evident arrhythmias or conduction abnormalities prior to sarcoidosis-related sudden death are often evident, if the appropriate screening takes place. It should be emphasized that sudden death can occur in the absence of a previous cardiac event as the primary event [17]!

Pearls of Wisdom
1. Cardiac Sarcoidosis remains highly prevalent in African Americans, almost three times the annual incidence of Caucasian Americans (35.5 cases per 100,000, as compared with 10.9 per 100,000). The lifetime risk of sarcoidosis in African Americans in the United States is quoted at approximately 2.4 %, compared with a lifetime risk of 0.85 % in Caucasians.
2. The highest reported incidence occurs in northern European countries and is quoted at 5–40 cases per 100,000 people.
3. Overall, the disease prevalence is estimated at 20 per 100,000.
4. For most cases, sarcoidosis develops before middle age, usually before age 50, with peak incidence in early adulthood, ages 20–39.
5. Sarcoidosis can involve nearly any organ system, but is most often found involving the pulmonary system in more than 90 % of the cases reported.
6. Clinical evidence of myocardial involvement is present in only about 5 % of patients with sarcoidosis. However, autopsy studies indicate that subclinical cardiac involvement is present in 20–30 % of cases.

References

1. Boeck C. Multiple benign sarcoid of the skin. J Cutan Genitourin Dis. 1899;17:543–50.
2. Hutchinson J. On eruptions which occur in connection with gout: case of Mortimer's malady. Arch Surg. 1898;9:307–14.
3. Hutchinson J. Case of livid papillary psoriasis. In: Illustrations of clinical surgery, vol. 1. London: J&A Churchill; 1877. p. 42–3.
4. Rybicki BA, Major M, Popovich Jr J, Maliarik MJ, Iannuzzi MC. Racial differences in sarcoidosis incidence: a 5-year study in a health maintenance organization. Am J Epidemiol. 1997;145:234–41.
5. Pietinalho A, Hiraga Y, Hosoda Y, L.froos AB, Yamaguchi M, Selroos O. The frequency of sarcoidosis in Finland and Hokkaido, Japan: a comparative epidemiological study. Sarcoidosis. 1995;12:61–7.
6. Thomas KW, Hunninghake GW. Sarcoidosis. JAMA. 2003;289:3300.
7. Baughman RP, Teirstein AS, Judson MA, et al. Clinical characteristics of patients in a case control study of sarcoidosis. Am J Respir Crit Care Med. 2001;164:1885–9.
8. Milman N, Selroos O. Pulmonary sarcoidosis in the Nordic countries 1950–1982: epidemiology and clinical picture. Sarcoidosis. 1990;7:50–7.
9. Iannuzzi MC, Rybicki BA, Teirstein AS. Sarcoidosis. N Engl J Med. 2007;357:2153–65.
10. Rabin DL, Thompson B, Brown KM, et al. Sarcoidosis: social predictors of severity at presentation. Eur Respir J. 2004;24:601–8.
11. Kim JS, Judson MA, Donnino R, et al. Cardiac sarcoidosis. Am Heart J. 2009;157:9.
12. Mehta D, Lubitz SA, Frankel Z, Wisnivesky JP, Einstein AJ, Goldman M, Machac J, Teirstein A. Cardiac involvement in patients with sarcoidosis: diagnostic and prognostic value of outpatient testing. Chest. 2008;133:1426–35.
13. Smedema JP, et al. Cardiac involvement in patients with pulmonary sarcoidosis assessed at two university medical centers in the Netherlands. Chest. 2005;128:30.
14. Iwai K, Sekiguti M, Hosoda Y, DeRemee RA, Tazelaar HD, Sharma OP, Maheshwari A, Noguchi TI. 1YY4. Racial difference in cardiac sarcoidosis incidence observed at autopsy. Sarcoidosis. 1994;11:26–31.
15. Yigla M, Badarna-Abu-Ria N, Tov N, et al. Sarcoidosis in northern Israel; clinical characteristics of 120 patients. Sarcoidosis Vasc Diffuse Lung Dis. 2002;19:220.
16. Soejima K, et al. The work-up and management of patients with apparent or subclinical cardiac sarcoidosis: with emphasis on the associated heart rhythm abnormalities. J Cardiovasc Electrophysiol. 2009;20:578.
17. Reuhl J, et al. Myocardial sarcoidosis as a rare cause of sudden cardiac death. Forensic Sci Int. 1997;89:145.

Chapter 2
Pathophysiology: From Genetics to Viruses and More

Andrew M. Freeman

Abstract Sarcoidosis is thought to occur in patients with some sort of genetic susceptibility in combination with an environmental exposure. The exact mechanisms are multifactorial and unclear, despite numerous leads explored over the years. Genetic foci, viruses, fungi, and environmental toxins have all been shown to be potentially involved in the development of the disease. Cardiac sarcoidosis develops as noncaseating granulomas which may involve the left ventricular free wall, basal ventricular septum, right ventricle, papillary muscles, right atrium, and left atrium. Cardiac involvement occurs in 20–27 % of sarcoidosis patients in the United States and may be as high as 58 % in Japan.

The Complicated Origins of Sarcoidosis

Sarcoidosis is thought to occur in patients with some sort of genetic susceptibility in combination with an environmental exposure, the so-called "two-hit" hypothesis. In this scenario, while one may have the genetic predisposition for the disease, it usually takes some environmental trigger, i.e. exposure, virus, or other to trigger the disease phenotype. This may help to explain the variable incidence throughout the world, as exposures, viruses, and other environmental variable are also quite varied among different populations.

The National Institutes of Health funded the multi-center ACCESS study (A Case-Control Etiologic Sarcoidosis Study) that investigated more than 700 patients and almost 30,000 relatives in an effort to identify the causative agent(s) for sarcoidosis, but unfortunately, no single agent or genetic locus was found to be responsible [1]. However, many potential leads into the causality of the disease were discovered.

There are some familial clusters of sarcoidosis known which is felt to be a genetic component with linkage to a section within major histocompatibility complex (MHC)

A.M. Freeman, MD, FACC, FACP
Division of Cardiology, Department of Medicine, National Jewish Health,
1400 Jackson St., Denver, CO 80206, USA
e-mail: freemana@njhealth.org

on the short arm of chromosome six. Familial clusters can occur with a rate of at least 19 % in African American families and only 5 % in Caucasian families. Monozygotic twins are more commonly affected than dizygotic twins [2]. Several alleles appear to confer susceptibility to disease (HLA DR 11, 12, 14, 15, 17) and others seem to be protective (e.g., HLA DRI, DR4, and possibly DQ*0202) [3]. Multiple serologic studies have identified primary associations with class I HLA-A1 and B8 and class II HLA-DR3 in Caucasians [4] In the ACCESS study described above, which included over 700 patients, over 27,000 first- and second-degree relatives were studies. ACCESS demonstrated increased risk in first-degree relatives for the development of sarcoidosis (odds ratio 4.7, 95 % CI 2.3–9.7). This risk was even greater for relatives of Caucasian patients than for African American patients (OR 18.0 versus 2.8) [1]

As of this publication, two human genome scans for loci associated with sarcoidosis have been completed. One study of Caucasian Germans, demonstrated strong association with chromosomes 3p and 6p [5], while the other study conducted in African Americans discovered the strongest signals at chromosomes 5p and 5q [6]. As one could imagine, outcomes of genome scans tend to be influenced by the populations studied.

Angiotensin-converting enzyme (ACE) genes have also been implicated, possibly suggesting why African Americans might be more afflicted by this disease process [7]. However, there is still no clear linkage between this genetic locus and causality of sarcoidosis. As a diagnostic tool, serum ACE measurements lack sensitivity and specificity. In one study, the positive and negative predictive values were only 84 and 74 %, respectively [8].

In delving deeper into genetics, T-cell makeup has been studied extensively. Lymphocytes inside of sarcoidosis granulomas are typically CD4+ T cells, while peripheral T cells are also CD4+ with CD8+ T cells [9]. When bronchoalveolar lavage has been performed in sarcoidosis patients, the aspirate shows increases in cellularity whereas periphery shows relative lymphopenia. Finally, CD1d-restricted natural killer cells (CD1d-rNKT cells), are decreased or absent in both the peripheral blood and BAL fluid, regardless of disease activity [10]. Many groups have also studied T-cell receptors with definitive etiology in the pathogenesis of sarcoidosis confirmed [11].

Along with T-cell and T-cell receptor pathology, there have been several reports of common variable immunodeficiency concurrent with cases of sarcoidosis in the literature. A 1996 series found 8 cases of common variable immunodeficiency (CVID) out of 80 patients with sarcoidosis and noted that 22 other cases had been reported in the literature [12].

Vitamin D receptor polymorphisms have been reported in Japanese patients with sarcoidosis [13]. Along with the vitamin D and calcium regulation pathways, calcitriol is often a key player in the disease state. As calcitriol has been found to be produced by activated pulmonary macrophages, derailment of calcium homeostasis often accompanies the sarcoidosis disease state. While, the significance of calcitriol in the pathogenesis of sarcoidosis is not known, it is in part responsible for the hypercalciuria and hypercalcemia that are frequently encountered clinically, and may even be implicated in nephrolithiasis that often accompanies these disease states (Table 2.1).

Table 2.1 Potential etiologies of sarcoidosis

Genetics: chromosomal abnormalities, angiotensin-converting enzyme genes
T cell abnormalities
T cell receptor abnormalities
Vitamin D receptor gene abnormalities
Viruses: HHV
Mycobacterial diseases and acid-fast cell wall-deficient organisms
Beryllium exposure
Humidity/water damage exposure
Propionibacterium
Common variable immunodeficiency
Other environmental exposures
Fungal infections/exposures

Table 2.2 Differential diagnosis of sarcoidosis

Mycobacterial infection
Fungal infection
Beryllium lung disease
Hypersensitivity pneumonitis HP
Wegener's granulomatosis
Collagen vascular disease
Lymphoma
Other infections
Drug/toxins

Since sarcoidosis is most often found in organs the directly interface to the environment (skin, eyes, lungs), it has been hypothesized that an environmental or toxic trigger would be found to cause the disease. Only beryllium salts (seen often at the author's institution in Denver, Colorado where beryllium mining is common) have been noted to create granulomas similar in appearance to those of sarcoidosis [14]. Another environmental exposure has also recently been identified. In this report, exposure to high humidity workplaces or water damage in association with a genetic susceptibility with the HLA-DQB1 locus has been found to be potentially causative in sarcoidosis [15].

In the 1960s, Dr. Siltzbach and colleagues created the Kviem-Siltzbach antigen, a derivative from human sarcoidosis tissue samples, which when injected intra-dermally, was able to create granulomatous inflammation for 70 % of patients for about 6 weeks [16]. Further studies of this antigen did not demonstrate definitive causality of this agent (Table 2.2).

Much attention has been given to pathologic organisms such as viruses, bacteria, and mycobacterial diseases. For mycobacteria, a number of studies, including those using hybridization techniques and PCR, have found evidence of *M. tuberculosis* in sarcoidosis tissue. Unfortunately, as mycobacteria are notoriously difficult to culture, these results have not been easily reproduced [17]. One particularly important study demonstrated the growth of acid-fast cell wall-deficient forms of bacteria sources from blood samples of 19 of 20 patients with sarcoidosis, which did not grow in the 20 controls [18]. Further analysis of these isolated organisms stained positively with an antibody raised against M. tuberculosis. Unfortunately, it was not possible to determine if these organisms were causative. A large case-control study subsequently found no clear differences in the cell walls of organisms in the blood of sarcoidosis patients [19].

One more common organism, responsible for acne in many populations, *propionibacterium*, has been thought to be involved in sarcoidosis pathogenesis. This organism is now considered to possibly activate the immune system to create the environment to develop sarcoidosis [20].

Viruses have also been given some of the blame for the development of sarcoidosis. Most notably, human herpes virus 8 has been implicated, particularly in lung biopsies of afflicted patients [21]. Unfortunately, no other studies looking at this herpes etiology could confirm these findings [22].

An interesting pilot study from 2007 reported the empiric use of anti-fungal drugs combined with corticosteroids for up to 6 months in 18 patients resulted in improvement of clinical symptoms, chest X-ray imaging, and pulmonary function testing [23]. This is has not yet been replicated.

In short, much work has been completed into the etiologic search for sarcoidosis without any clear pathway to disease development. Ultimately, future immunogenetic research will likely yield more answers. Until then, continued screening, evaluation, and keeping sarcoidosis on the differential is critical to discovering those patients who have the disease but who may otherwise go unrecognized, with often dire consequences.

The clinical manifestations of sarcoidosis are dependent on both the development and location of granulomas. Cardiac sarcoidosis develops as noncaseating granulomas which may involve the left ventricular free wall, basal ventricular septum, right ventricle, papillary muscles, right atrium, and left atrium develop [24]. Histopathology of cardiac sarcoidosis suggests three successive stages: edema, granulomatous infiltration, and fibrosis and scar formation. Biopsy pathology demonstrates the presence of numerous lymphocytes in the border zones around the granulomas with a dense band of fibroblasts, collagen fibers, and proteoglycans which encircle an aggregate of inflammatory cells [24].

Cardiac involvement occurs in 20–27 % of sarcoidosis patients in the United States and may be as high as 58 % in Japan [25]. The prevalence of cardiac findings in cardiac sarcoidosis is variable and includes complete heart block, bundle branch block, ventricular tachycardia, congestive heart failure, and sudden cardiac death most commonly (12–75 % of the time) [2].

Pearls of Wisdom
1. Sarcoidosis is thought to occur in patients with some sort of genetic susceptibility in combination with an environmental exposure, the so-called "two-hit" hypothesis.
2. The National Institutes of Health funded the multi-center ACCESS study (A Case-Control Etiologic Sarcoidosis Study) that investigated more than 700 patients and almost 30,000 relatives in an effort to identify the causative agent(s) for sarcoidosis, but unfortunately, no single agent or genetic locus was found to be responsible.
3. Genetic loci have been found to be linked to cases of sarcoidosis in some populations.
4. Potential causes for the disease include viral infections, fungal infections, bacterial infection, humidity, and environmental toxins.
5. Histopathology of cardiac sarcoidosis suggests three successive stages: edema, granulomatous infiltration, and fibrosis and scar formation.

References

1. Rybicki BA, Iannuzzi MC, Frederick MM, et al. Familial aggregation of sarcoidosis. A case-control etiologic study of sarcoidosis (ACCESS). Am J Respir Crit Care Med. 2001;164:2085.
2. Sekhri V, et al. Cardiac sarcoidosis: a comprehensive review. Arch Med Sci. 2011;7(4): 546–54.
3. Baughman RP, Lower EE, du Bois RM. Sarcoidosis. Lancet. 2003;361:1111.
4. Lee LS, Rose CS, Maier LA. Sarcoidosis. N Engl J Med. 1997;336:1224–34.
5. Schurmann M, Reichel P, Muller-Myhsok B, Schlaak M, Muller-Quernheim J, Schwinger E. Results from a genome-wide search for predisposing genes in sarcoidosis. Am J Respir Crit Care Med. 2001;164:840–6.
6. Iannuzzi MC, Iyengar SK, Gray-McGuire C, et al. Genome-wide search for sarcoidosis susceptibility genes in African Americans. Genes Immun. 2005;6:509–18.
7. Maliarik MJ, Rybicki BA, Malvitz E, et al. Angiotensin-converting enzyme gene polymorphism and risk of sarcoidosis. Am J Respir Crit Care Med. 1998;158:1566.
8. Studdy PR, Bird R. Serum angiotensin converting enzyme in sarcoidosis—its value in present clinical practice. Ann Clin Biochem. 1989;26:13–8.
9. Semenzato G, Pezzutto A, Chilosi M, Pizzolo G. Redistribution of T lymphocytes in the lymph nodes of patients with sarcoidosis. N Engl J Med. 1982;306:48.
10. Ho LP, Urban BC, Thickett DR, et al. Deficiency of a subset of T-cells with immunoregulatory properties in sarcoidosis. Lancet. 2005;365:1062.
11. Moller DR, Konishi K, Kirby M, et al. Bias toward use of a specific T cell receptor beta-chain variable region in a subgroup of individuals with sarcoidosis. J Clin Invest. 1988;82:1183.

12. Fasano MB, Sullivan KE, Sarpong SB, et al. Sarcoidosis and common variable immunodeficiency. Report of 8 cases and review of the literature. Medicine (Baltimore). 1996;75:251.
13. Niimi T, Tomita H, Sato S, et al. Vitamin D receptor gene polymorphism in patients with sarcoidosis. Am J Respir Crit Care Med. 1999;160:1107.
14. Moller DR, Chen ES. What causes sarcoidosis? Curr Opin Pulm Med. 2002;8:429.
15. Iannuzzi MC, Maliarik MJ, Poisson LM, Rybicki BA. Sarcoidosis susceptibility and resistance HLA-DQB1 alleles in African Americans. Am J Respir Crit Care Med. 2003;167:1225–31.
16. Siltzbach LE. The Kveim test in sarcoidosis. A study of 750 patients. JAMA. 1961;178:476.
17. Mitchell IC, Turk JL, Mitchell DN. Detection of mycobacterial rRNA in sarcoidosis with liquid-phase hybridisation. Lancet. 1992;339:1015.
18. Almenoff PL, Johnson A, Lesser M, Mattman LH. Growth of acid fast L forms from the blood of patients with sarcoidosis. Thorax. 1996;51:530.
19. Brown ST, Brett I, Almenoff PL, et al. Recovery of cell wall-deficient organisms from blood does not distinguish between patients with sarcoidosis and control subjects. Chest. 2003;123:413.
20. Nishiwaki T, Yoneyama H, Eishi Y, et al. Indigenous pulmonary Propionibacterium acnes primes the host in the development of sarcoid-like pulmonary granulomatosis in mice. Am J Pathol. 2004;165:631.
21. Di Alberti L, Piattelli A, Artese L, et al. Human herpesvirus 8 variants in sarcoid tissues. Lancet. 1997;350:1655.
22. Bélec L, Mohamed AS, Lechapt-Zalcman E, et al. Lack of HHV-8 DNA sequences in sarcoid tissues of French patients. Chest. 1998;114:948.
23. Tercelj M, Rott T, Rylander R. Antifungal treatment in Sarcoidosis a pilot intervention trial. Respir Med. 2007;101:774–8.
24. Roberts WC, McAllister HA, Ferrans VJ. Sarcoidosis of the heart A clinicopathologic study of 35 necropsy patients (group I) and review of 78 previously described necropsy patients (group II). Am J Med. 1977;63:86–108.
25. Matsui Y, Iwai K, Tachibana T, et al. Clinicopathological study on fatal myocardial sarcoidosis. Ann N Y Acad Sci. 1976;278:455–69.

Chapter 3
Clinical Presentations

Howard D. Weinbeger

Abstract Cardiac sarcoidosis is a true chameleon of disease in that it can present like many other cardiac and pulmonary conditions and hide the true etiology of sarcoidosis. Manifestations can be as mild as asymptomatic first degree AV block to the more severe and potentially lethal ventricular arrhythmia or high degree heart block, severe valvular disease or cardiomyopathy and heart failure. There is no standard or routine test for cardiac sarcoidosis and its diagnosis depends on an expert team, a careful history and physical, and appropriate testing.

Cardiac sarcoidosis may present symptomatically in several different ways, may present with relatively non-specific symptoms, or may be identified in an asymptomatic individual. The true incidence of cardiac involvement is difficult to determine due to the lack of a highly sensitive and specific "gold standard" test, as well as the apparent differences from country to country. For example, in the United States 13–25 % of deaths in patients with sarcoidosis are due to cardiac sarcoidosis while in Japan 47–85 % of deaths in patients with sarcoidosis are due to cardiac sarcoidosis. Because of these and other limitations, cardiac sarcoidosis is likely under diagnosed. Most studies report an incidence of ~5 % while autopsy studies suggest up to 70 % of patients with sarcoidosis have cardiac involvement [1]. Unfortunately, the first clinical manifestation of cardiac sarcoidosis may be sudden cardiac death or a life threatening conduction abnormality or arrhythmia. This underscores the importance of considering and looking for evidence of cardiac involvement in patients with sarcoidosis before a serious or life threatening complication occurs.

Clinically symptomatic presentations include conduction abnormalities such as complete heart block and syncope, AV block, bundle branch block, tachyarrhythmias (classically ventricular arrhythmias, and more recent appreciation that atrial arrhythmias may be the first indication of cardiac sarcoidosis) [2], ventricular and

---

H.D. Weinbeger, MD, FACC, FACP
Division of Cardiology, Department of Medicine, National Jewish Health,
1400 Jackson St., Denver, CO 80206, USA
e-mail: weinbergerh@njhealth.org

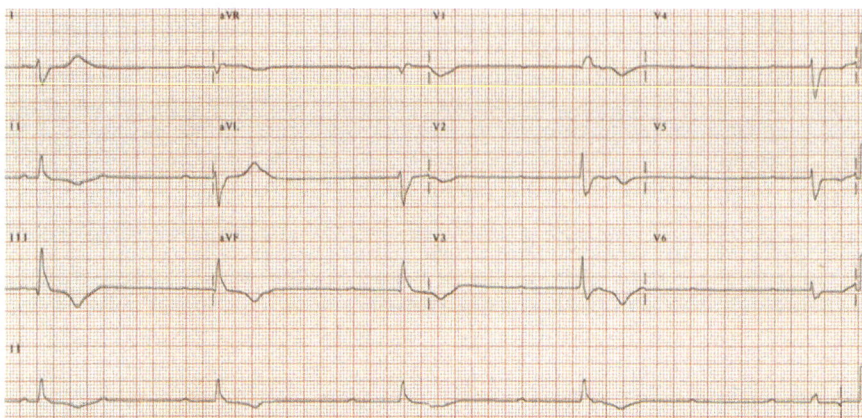

Fig. 3.1 Complete heart block

atrial ectopy, cardiomyopathy, congestive heart failure, sudden cardiac death, valvular dysfunction, coronary artery vasculitis, and pericardial disease.

Complete heart block has been reported as the most common clinical presentation of cardiac sarcoidosis, and occurs at a younger age than those that have complete heart block from non-cardiac sarcoidosis causes [1, 3, 4]. Ventricular tachycardia, both sustained and non-sustained and frequent ventricular ectopy are the second most common clinical presentation of cardiac sarcoidosis [1]. Both heart block (Fig. 3.1) and ventricular arrhythmias may cause syncope, which may be the initial presentation.

Cardiac sarcoidosis may be mis-diagnosed as arrhythmogenic right ventricular cardiomyopathy (ARVC) [1, 5–7]. Cardiac sarcoidosis should be considered in patients with non-ischemic cardiomyopathy, left ventricular systolic dysfunction and congestive heart failure. Congestive heart failure is the second most common cause of death, following sudden cardiac death, in patients with cardiac sarcoidosis.

Valvular dysfunction most often involves the mitral valve, and is more commonly due to papillary muscle dysfunction as a result of myocardial involvement (Fig. 3.2). Pericardial effusion may occur, and the first reported case of cardiac sarcoidosis was that of pericardial granulomas [8].

Patients with cardiac sarcoidosis may present with a variety of non-specific symptoms including palpitations, chest pain, and dyspnea. The electrocardiogram may be abnormal in up to 50 % of patients with sarcoidosis without clinically evident cardiac involvement [1, 4]. These abnormalities may be mild and non-specific such as a fragmented QRS complex, atrio-ventricular block or bundle branch block [9, 10]. A patient with sarcoidosis and possible cardiac related symptoms or any abnormality on the electrocardiogram should under go further evaluation for cardiac sarcoidosis.

Because there is no "gold standard" test for cardiac sarcoidosis and serious or life threatening complications may be the initial clinical presentation, keeping a high index of suspicion and a low threshold to pursue evaluation for possible cardiac involvement in patients with sarcoidosis is imperative.

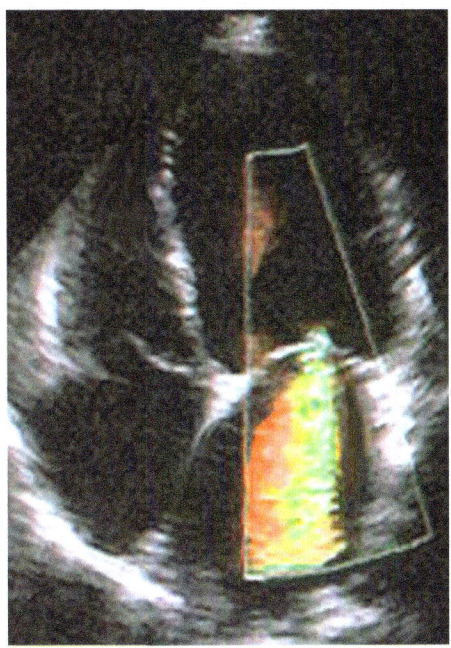

Fig. 3.2 Severe mitral regurgitation in a 56 year old sarcoidosis patient

Pearls of Wisdom
1. There is no gold standard test for cardiac sarcoidosis.
2. Clinical presentations vary from no clinically noticeable symptoms to marked dyspnea, syncope, fatigue and more.
3. The first manifestation of cardiac sarcoidosis can be sudden cardiac death.

References

1. Bargout R, Kelly RF. Sarcoid heart disease: clinical course and treatment. Int J Cardiol. 2004;97:173.
2. Viles-Gonzales JF, Pastori L, Fischer A, et al. Supraventricular arrhythmias in patients with cardiac sarcoidosis: prevalence, predictors and clinical implications. Chest. 2013;143:1085.
3. Chapelon-Abric C, de Zuttere D, Duhaul P, et al. Cardiac sarcoidosis: a retrospective study of 41 cases. Medicine (Baltimore). 2004;83:315.
4. Sekhri V, Sanal S, DeLorenzo LJ, et al. Cardiac sarcoidosis: a comprehensive review. Arch Med Sci. 2011;7(4):546.
5. Mohsen A, Panday M, Wetherold S, et al. Cardiac sarcoidosis mimicking arrhythmogenic right ventricular dysplasia with high defibrillation threshold requiring subcutaneous shocking coil implantation. Heart Lung Circ. 2012;21:46.
6. Yared K, Johri AM, Soni AV, et al. Cardiac sarcoidosis imitating arrhythmogenic right ventricular dysplasia. Circulation. 2008;118:e113.
7. Chia PL, Subbiah RN, Kuchar D, et al. Cardiac sarcoidosis masquerading as arrhythmogenic right ventricular cardiomyopathy. Heart Lung Circ. 2012;21:42.

8. Bernstein M, Konglemann FW, Sidlick DM. Boeck's sarcoid. Report of a case with visceral involvement. Arch Intern Med. 1929;44:721–34.
9. Zipse MM, Sauer WH. Electrophysiologic manifestations of cardiac sarcoidosis. Curr Opin Pulm Med. 2013;19:485.
10. Homsi M, Alsayed L, Safadi B, et al. Fragmented QRS complexes on 12-lead ECG: a marker of cardiac sarcoidosis as detected by gadolinium cardiac magnetic resonance imaging. Ann Noninvasive Electrocardiol. 2009;14(4):319.

Chapter 4
Standard Screening for Cardiac Sarcoidosis

Andrew M. Freeman

Abstract Arrhythmia, heart failure, valvular dysfunction, heart block, pericardial disease, and sudden cardiac death are just some of the potential manifestations of cardiac sarcoidosis. A high clinical index of suspicion and regular surveillance in appropriate individuals is an important clinical management philosophy. Unfortunately, the severity of pulmonary disease does not predict cardiac involvement, and cardiac involvement can often present after pulmonary improvement. Electrocardiography, echocardiography, signal-averaged ECG, ambulatory telemetry monitoring, and cardiac magnetic resonance imaging are all helpful in the diagnosis and surveillance of cardiac sarcoidosis. Ambulatory monitoring has emerged as one of the more powerful tools to detect cardiac involvement, though an emerging composite scoring system may help even further.

Screening

Cardiac sarcoidosis is one of the most feared manifestations of the sarcoidosis disease complex. Arrhythmia, heart failure, valvular dysfunction, heart block, pericardial disease, and sudden cardiac death are just some of the potential manifestations of the disease. A high clinical index of suspicion and regular surveillance in appropriate individuals is of the utmost importance. As previously mentioned, cardiac sarcoidosis can have its first manifestation be sudden cardiac death. As such, timely diagnosis before a lethal complication presents is critical.

It is imperative that clinicians caring for sarcoidosis patients recognize that cardiac involvement may precede, follow, or occur simultaneously with pulmonary involvement or other organs. In an analysis of 52 patients with cardiac sarcoidosis from Germany, about one-third of the cases cardiac involvement became apparent after the lung changes had already normalized [1]. The severity of pulmonary

---

A.M. Freeman, MD, FACC, FACP
Division of Cardiology, Department of Medicine, National Jewish Health,
1400 Jackson St., Denver, CO 80206, USA
e-mail: freemana@njhealth.org

Table 4.1 Japanese Ministry of Health criteria for cardiac sarcoidosis

Histologic diagnosis
Endomyocardial biopsy demonstrating noncaseating epithelioid granulomas
Clinical diagnosis
Suspect cardiac sarcoidosis with (a) + one other
(a) Complete right bundle branch block, AV block, ventricular tachycardia, ventricular premature beats or pathologic Q wave or ST-T changes on the electrocardiogram
(b) Abnormal wall motion, regional wall thickening, or left ventricular dilation
(c) Perfusion defect on myocardial perfusion imaging or abnormal accumulation of 67-Gallium citrate or 99mTc-PYP myocardial scintigraphy
(d) Abnormal intracardiac pressure, low cardiac output, or abnormal wall motion or reduced ejection fraction of the left ventricle
(e) On endomyocardial biopsy, interstitial fibrosis or more than moderate cellular infiltration, even if the findings are nonspecific

Adapted from Hiraga et al. [3]

disease does not predict cardiac involvement [2]. In short, a healthcare provider should always be on the lookout for cardiac sarcoidosis, even when the lung disease is quiescent.

There is no gold standard for the diagnosis of cardiac sarcoidosis. Guidelines for diagnosing cardiac sarcoidosis have been published by the Japanese Ministry of Health and Welfare (JMHW) and are frequently referenced and followed in making the diagnosis of cardiac sarcoidosis [3]. However, it is not clear if these guidelines are generalizable to other groups (Table 4.1).

Cardiac magnetic resonance imaging (cMRI) and cardiac 18-flourodeoxuyglucose positron emission tomography (FDG-cPET) are being utilized as noninvasive diagnostic tests of choice for cardiac sarcoidosis. However, both cMRI and FDG-cPET are expensive, not readily available, and are likely not the best choice for routine screening.

In this chapter, we will review screening for cardiac sarcoidosis using the more readily available clinical tools of electrocardiography, signal-averaged ECG, ambulatory monitoring, and echocardiography.

Electrocardiography

Simple, inexpensive, and readily available characterize electrocardiography (ECG). Unfortunately, due to the short time frame of sampling with ECG, many findings may be missed, especially intermittent conduction disease. Complete heart block is the most common finding in patients with clinically evident cardiac sarcoidosis. Heart block often occurs at a younger age in patients with sarcoidosis than in individuals with complete heart block due to other etiologies [4]. First-degree AV block (PR prolongation) due to atrio-ventricular nodal disease or bundle of His, and other

4 Standard Screening for Cardiac Sarcoidosis

intraventricular conduction diseases are frequently seen [5]. It is important to note that most of these issues may initially be silent but can often rapidly progress to complete heart block, marked bradycardia, and syncope. A low threshold to perform an ECG at a moment's notice should be part of the clinical toolbox available to sarcoidosis patients without currently known cardiac involvement.

As the sarcoidosis disease process develops, granulomas can develop in almost any tissue. As they develop in the heart, substrate for arrhythmia is created in that granulomas can effectively block or redirect conduction. Since granulomas develop into scar, they do not conduct electrical impulses, and can create islands of non-conducting tissue that have the potential to develop arrhythmia. Areas of active inflammation may also create areas of automaticity leading to re-entrant dysrhythmias. Ventricular arrhythmias are the second most common presentation of cardiac sarcoidosis. This includes both sustained and non-sustained ventricular tachycardias. As many as 22 % of patients with sarcoidosis may demonstrate ventricular arrhythmia on ECG [6].

In clinical practice, and in the electrophysiology realm (see Chaps. 8, 9, and 12), atrial sarcoidosis has been described creating virtually any atrial dysrhythmia such as atrial fibrillation, atrial flutter, and atrial tachycardia.

In any person with otherwise unexplained ventricular arrhythmia, heart block, or conduction disease, a search for sarcoidosis involving the conduction system should be part of the workup.

Signal-Averaged ECG

Signal Averaged ECG (SAECG) is a simple non-invasive electrocardiographic test that detects low amplitude signals at the end of the QRS complex that are known as "late potentials" [7]. SAECG has been used clinically to identify patients at increased risk of ventricular arrhythmias [8] after myocardial infarction or with arrhythmogenic right ventricular dysplasia. In one study, SAECG was abnormal in 46 % of patients with pulmonary sarcoidosis with no clinical evidence of cardiac sarcoidosis [9]. The presence or absence of cardiac sarcoidosis was not confirmed by imaging modalities in that study.

A recent study by Schuller et al. [10] evaluated patients with suspected cardiac sarcoidosis as defined by Japanese Ministry of Health criteria and/or delayed gadolinium contrast enhancement on cardiac MRI. In this study, they found 27 of 88 patients included had cardiac sarcoidosis based on JMHW criteria with MRI. The authors found the sensitivity of SAECG detection of cardiac sarcoidosis was 52 % with a specificity of 82 %. In addition, they calculated a positive predictive value (PPV) of 0.56 and a negative predictive value (NPV) of 0.79. Within a subgroup of the 67 patients with an unfiltered QRS duration of <100 ms, they found the specificity for diagnosing cardiac sarcoidosis improves to 100 % with a reduced sensitivity of 36.8 % (Table 4.2).

Table 4.2 Criteria for abnormal signal averaged ECGs

Criteria used for establishing positive signal-averaged ECG
1. Noise must be less than 0.3 to be interpretable
2. Filtered QRS: ≤124 ms in males; ≤116 ms in females
3. HFLA/LAS: ≤42 ms in males and females
4. Root Mean Square (RMS): ≥16 in males; ≥15 in females
Items 2–4 above are the domains and the number of abnormal domains over the denominator of 3 should be reported

Echocardiography

In sarcoidosis patients without an obvious cause for heart failure, cardiac sarcoidosis rises to the top of the differential diagnosis. Echocardiography makes it easy assess ventricular function as well as any potential valvular involvement or wall motion abnormality. In patients with other known cardiac abnormalities such as those found in the conduction system, echocardiography should be performed.

In a study by Burstow et al. echocardiographic changes were detected in 14 % of patients with systemic sarcoidosis, but in another 11 %, echocardiogram was within normal limits although there were significant clinically unexplained conduction abnormalities likely related to sarcoidosis [11].

Possible abnormalities seen on echocardiography include left ventricular cavity enlargement, septal wall thinning (particularly of the basal segment) or segmental wall motion abnormalities of the left ventricle, left ventricular aneurysm, valvular regurgitation. Also possible is mitral valve prolapse, but this is not specific to cardiac sarcoidosis involvement. Right ventricular dilatation and hypokinesis can be seen as well, particularly with extensive pulmonary involvement, and with development of pulmonary hypertension. There are several reports of hyperechoic (commonly referred to as "sparkling") signal of the left ventricular myocardium when there is granulomatous involvement and scar formation [12] (Fig. 4.1).

Sarcoidosis lesions of the myocardium may show up with an increased myocardial wall thickness, simulating left ventricular hypertrophy, or increased interventricular septal thickness, resembling hypertrophic cardiomyopathy.

If wall motion abnormalities are present from cardiac sarcoidosis, they usually do not follow typical coronary distributions. It is of course certainly possible to have coexistent coronary disease, and ischemia should be sought as a cause of wall motion abnormalities in appropriate individuals.

Pulmonary hypertension, described in Chap. 13, is often detected with echocardiography in patients with pulmonary hypertension. In these cases, elevated right ventricular systolic pressure in the setting of right heart dysfunction often suggests this disease process. This diagnosis must be confirmed with directly measured values via a right heart catheterization. The World Health Organization classifies this as group V pulmonary hypertension (pulmonary hypertension due to underlying systemic diseases).

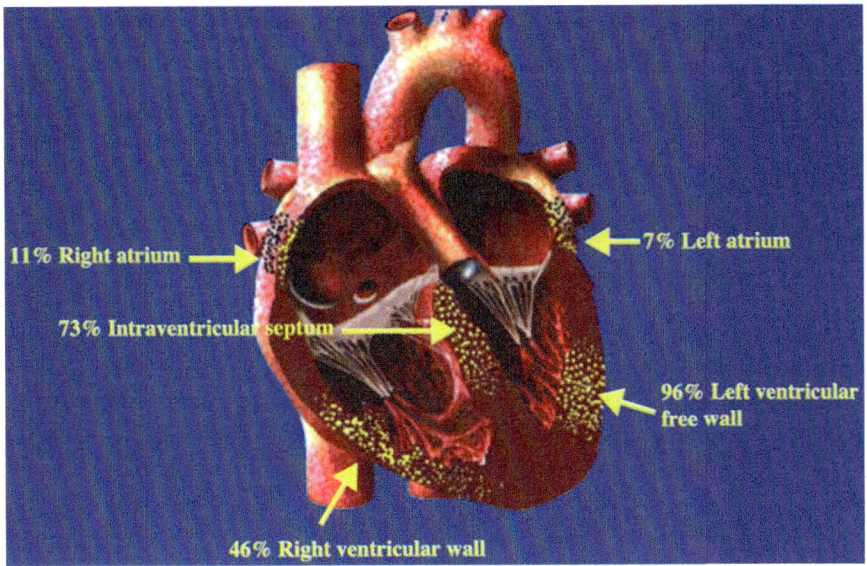

Fig. 4.1 Likely locations of cardiac sarcoidosis involvement (From Bargout and Kelly [18] with permission)

Ambulatory Electrocardiographic Monitoring

Ambulatory electrocardiographic monitoring, most often known as Holter or mobile telemetry monitoring, reduces the problem of too short of a sampling period with a standard ECG. Using either 24 or 48 h monitoring, clinicians can determine not only if there is a conduction defect, but can also significantly monitor the burden of arrhythmia, ventricular ectopy, and even evaluate for atrial arrhythmias, Ambulatory ECG monitoring has proven itself as the most useful of the non-imaging modalities [2].

In a small study of 38 patients [13] with systemic sarcoidosis referred for cardiologic evaluation, 7 of 12 patients (67 %) with confirmed cardiac sarcoidosis had >100 premature ventricular contractions per day as compared to only 8 % of the 26 patients without cardiac sarcoidosis. In that study, only 5 % of 58 healthy controls had this degree of ventricular ectopy. This study demonstrated that Holter monitoring has a sensitivity of 67 % and a specificity of 80 % [13].

Many centers use Holter monitoring as part of the yearly surveillance of patients with sarcoidosis, as it represents a very inexpensive yet thorough assessment of the cardiac conduction system. It has also been the basis for many ICD implants, in that non-sustained ventricular tachycardia detected on such a device often necessitates additional workup such as electrophysiology study, advanced imaging such as cardiac MRI to determine scar burden, and more.

Sudden cardiac death (SCD) due to ventricular tachyarrhythmias or serious conduction block accounts for up to 65 % of deaths due to cardiac sarcoidosis [14]. While many patients with known systemic sarcoidosis develop symptomatic conduction disease on electrocardiogram prior to sarcoidosis-related sudden death, many patients do not. It is important to underscore the understanding that sudden cardiac death (SCD) can occur in the absence of symptoms or a previous cardiac event [15].

A Word About Endomyocardial Biopsy

While one would think that tissue diagnosis is the best for many enigmatic diseases, cardiac sarcoidosis is challenging to capture this way. Detection of non-caseating granulomas is indeed the "gold standard" for diagnosis of cardiac sarcoidosis but is often difficult to perform reliably owing to the patchy nature of the disease. This patchiness leaves islands of entirely normal tissue adjacent to significantly diseased granulomatous tissue. As such, a right heart catheterization with endomyocardial biopsy is prone to "missing" the areas of diseases tissue and is only recommended if the patient lacks histological confirmation of non-caseating granulomas from any other source.

As sarcoidosis experts will often recount, a right heart myocardial biopsy has a low sensitivity, sometimes quoted at around 20 % [16]. This may be significantly lower in those with normal ventricular function. Additionally, since myocardial granulomas tend to affect the basal and lateral left ventricular walls, these are often not biopsied due to the potential risk for serious complication such as stroke, perforation, embolus, or death (see a more in depth discussion of endomyocardial biopsy in Chap. 8).

Putting It All Together

As you have seen in this chapter, establishing the diagnosis of cardiac sarcoidosis by commonly available modalities is challenging. As the proliferation of advanced imaging studies such as cardiac MRI and cardiac 18-FDG-PET are still not widely available, making use of all available screening tools is essential.

While no modality is best, the highest yield modality is ambulatory ECG monitoring (Holter monitoring) and is recommended by the author as a screening tool in selected and appropriate individuals owing to low cost, ease of administration, and good results.

A recent study published in 2013 [17] by some of the authors of this book evaluated a scoring system (see Tables 4.3a and 4.3b) which was able to take all of the potential screening modalities a patient might undergo to help predict who might have a positive cardiac MRI or cardiac 18-flouro-deoxuyglucose positron emission tomography. In this study, sensitivity and specificity of the various modalities were also reported (see Table 4.4) The results indicated that combining all of the available

Table 4.3a Proposed cardiac sarcoidosis scoring criteria [17]

Criteria	Major	Minor
EKG/ambulatory monitoring	VT	Supraventricular arrhythmia
	2nd degree Type II	1st degree AV block
	3rd degree block	RBBB
		LBBB
		PVC
		Other atrioventricular block
		Conduction delays
SAECG		Each abnormal domain
Echocardiogram	LV systolic dysfunction (EF <55 %)	RV systolic dysfunction
		Wall motion abnormalities
		Wall thinning
		Diastolic dysfunction
EP study (if performed for a clinically indicated reason)	Monomorphic VT	Polymorphic VT
		Abnormal voltage mapping
		Conduction delays
Myocardial perfusion stress test		Reverse perfusion defect (stress images exhibit greater perfusion than rest)

Table 4.3b Proposed minor criteria score (per item listed) [17]

1 point	2 points	3 points
Diastolic dysfunction	Supraventricular arrhythmia	Abnormal voltage mapping
Wall thinning	LBBB	Conduction delays on EP study
RV dysfunction	Abnormal SAECG domain	
RBBB	Reverse SPECT perfusion defect (stress images exhibit greater perfusion than rest)	
1st Degree AV block		
Wall motion abnormalities		

LV left ventricle, *RV* right ventricle, *AV* atrioventricular, *VT* ventricular tachycardia, *EP* electrophysiology, *RBBB* right bundle branch block, *LBBB* left bundle branch block, *PVC* premature ventricular contraction

modalities correlated with the likelihood of a positive MRI or PET: A 1-point increase in total score increased the probability of positive cardiac MRI or cardiac 18-flouro-deoxuyglucose positron emission tomography by 14 % (P=0.01) [95 % CI: a 3–25 % increase]. The scoring system seemed to be driven more by cardiac MRI over cardiac 18-flouro-deoxuyglucose positron emission tomography: In patients who had cardiac MRI alone, for each 1-point increase in total score, the probability of positive cardiac MRI increases 11 % [95 % CI: a 1 % decrease – 25 % increase, P=0.08].

Table 4.4 Summary of diagnostic procedures' sensitivities and specificities for a positive imaging result (a positive cMRI or a positive FDG-cPET) [17]

Procedure	n	Sensitivity (%)	Specificity (%)	PPV	NPV
Echocardiography: any major or minor finding	64	62	29	60	32
Echocardiography: major finding (reduced LVEF)	32	32	70	70	32
Echocardiography: minor finding (RV systolic dysfunction, wall motion abnormalities, wall thinning, diastolic dysfunction)	54	55	33	56	32
ECG: minor finding[a]	55	58	55	66	46
ECG: VT or AV block	30	26	64	56	33
Ambulatory monitoring: any major or minor finding	47	89	21	62	57
Ambulatory monitoring: major finding	17	73	67	80	57
Ambulatory monitoring: minor finding	37	85	24	57	57
Signal averaged ECG: any abnormal domain	49	28	80	67	43
Nuclear stress testing	25	53	50	62	42
EP study	29	40	71	60	53

Sample sizes do not sum because negative findings were utilized to calculate PPV/NPV
FDG-cPET cardiac 18-flouro-deoxuyglucose positron emission tomography, *cMRI* cardiac magnetic resonance imaging, *ECG* electrocardiogram, *VT* ventricular tachycardia, *AV* atrio-ventricular, *EP* electrophysiology, *PPV* positive predictive value, *NPV* negative predictive value
[a]There were no major ECG findings in any subject

Pearls of Wisdom
1. Any cardiac structure can be involved in cardiac sarcoidosis.
2. Arrhythmia, heart failure, valvular dysfunction, heart block, pericardial disease, and sudden cardiac death are just some of the potential manifestations of cardiac sarcoidosis.
3. Regular surveillance may be appropriate in selected individuals.
4. Do not rely on lung function or lung involvement to decide when to screen for cardiac sarcoidosis.
5. Consider regular ECG and ambulatory ECG monitoring as they are low cost and readily available to help monitor for evidence of cardiac sarcoidosis.
6. Consider a composite scoring system to help predict which patients may have positive imaging and are more likely to have cardiac sarcoidosis.

References

1. Schaedel H, Kirsten D, Schmidt A, et al. Sarcoid heart disease – results of follow-up investigations. Eur Heart J. 1991;12(Suppl D):26.
2. Mehta D, Lubitz SA, Frankel Z, Wisnivesky JP, Einstein AJ, Goldman M, Machac J, Teirstein A. Cardiac involvement in patients with sarcoidosis: diagnostic and prognostic value of outpatient testing. Chest. 2008;133:1426–35.
3. Hiraga H, Hiroe M, Iwai K. Guideline for diagnosis of cardiac sarcoidosis: study report on diffuse pulmonary diseases. Tokyo: The Japanese Ministry of Health and Welfare; 1993. p. 23–4.
4. Fleming H. Cardiac sarcoidosis. In: James DG, editor. Sarcoidosis and other granulomatous disorders. New York: Dekker; 1994. p. 323.
5. Chapelon-Abric C, de Zuttere D, Duhaut P, et al. Cardiac sarcoidosis: a retrospective study of 41 cases. Medicine (Baltimore). 2004;83:315.
6. Yoshida Y, Morimoto S, Hiramitsu S, et al. Incidence of cardiac sarcoidosis in Japanese patients with high-degree atrioventricular block. Am Heart J. 1997;134:382.
7. Kunavarapu C, Bloomfield DM. Role of noninvasive studies in risk stratification for sudden cardiac death. Clin Cardiol. 2004;27(4):192–7.
8. Iravanian S, Arshad A, Steinberg JS. Role of electrophysiologic studies, signal-averaged electrocardiography, heart rate variability, T-wave alternans, and loop recorders for risk stratification of ventricular arrhythmias. Am J Geriatr Cardiol. 2005;14(1):16–9.
9. Yodogawa K, Seino Y, Ohara T, et al. Non-invasive detection of latent cardiac conduction abnormalities in patients with pulmonary sarcoidosis. Circ J. 2007;71(4):540–5.
10. Schuller JL, Lowery CM, Zipse M, Aleong RG, Varosy PD, Weinberger HD, Sauer WH. Diagnostic utility of signal averaged electrocardiography for detection of cardiac sarcoidosis. Ann Noninvasive Electrocardiol. 2011;16(1):70–6.
11. Burstow DJ, Tajik AJ, Bailey KR, DeRemee RA, Taliercio CP. Two-dimensional echocardiographic findings in systemic sarcoidosis. Am J Cardiol. 1989;63(7):478–82.
12. Sun BJ, Lee PH, Choi HO, et al. Prevalence of echocardiographic features suggesting cardiac sarcoidosis in patients with pacemaker or implantable cardiac defibrillator. Korean Circ J. 2011;41:313.
13. Suzuki T, Kanda T, Kubota S, et al. Holter monitoring as a noninvasive indicator of cardiac involvement in sarcoidosis. Chest. 1994;106:1021.
14. Schulte W, Kirsten D, Drent M, Costabel U. Cardiac involvement in sarcoidosis. Eur Respir Mon. 2005;32:130.
15. Patel MR, Cawley PJ, Heitner JF, et al. Detection of myocardial damage in patients with sarcoidosis. Circulation. 2009;120:1969.
16. Uemura A, Morimoto S, Hiramitsu S, et al. Histologic diagnostic rate of cardiac sarcoidosis: evaluation of endomyocardial biopsies. Am Heart J. 1999;138:299.
17. Freeman AM, Curran-Everett D, Weinberger HD, Fenster BE, Buckner JK, Gottschall EB, Hamzeh NY. Predictors of cardiac sarcoidosis using commonly available cardiac studies. Am J Cardiol. 2013;112(2):280–5.
18. Bargout R, Kelly RF. Sarcoid heart disease: clinical course and treatment. Intl J Card. 2004;97:173–82.

Chapter 5
Diagnosis II: Imaging of Cardiac Sarcoidosis with Cardiac MRI, PET and SPECT

Joyce D. Schroeder and Brett Fenster

Abstract Imaging protocols in Cardiac MRI, PET and SPECT provide a rich set of tools for the evaluation of myocardial scar, edema, inflammation, anatomy, functional abnormalities and associated features of cardiac sarcoidosis. Cardiac magnetic resonance imaging (MRI) employs delayed hyperenhancement (DHE) sequences for the detection of bright (high signal intensity) scar in the myocardium as well as T2 imaging for inflammation and cinematic movie imaging for anatomic and functional evaluation. PET/CT assesses for hypermetabolic inflammation within the myocardium using a PET protocol designed to suppress normal myocardial glucose uptake. Nuclear medicine Technetium (99mTc) sestamibi myocardial single-photon emission computed tomography (SPECT) assesses for "reverse distribution", perfusion abnormalities seen on rest imaging that are not present on stress imaging that may suggest microvascular constriction in myocardial sarcoidosis. However, Cardiac MRI, PET and SPECT imaging modalities are not individually specific for cardiac sarcoidosis and the role of imaging in the diagnosis and followup of cardiac sarcoidosis requires careful integration with laboratory and clinical data.

Role of Cardiac MRI in the Diagnosis of Cardiac Sarcoidosis

Cardiac magnetic resonance imaging (MRI) is a useful tool in the diagnosis of cardiac sarcoidosis primarily through the use of delayed hyperenhancement (DHE) sequences for the detection of bright (high signal intensity) scar in the myocardium. T2 weighted imaging is used for the detection of high signal intensity acute edema or inflammation. Although the detection of delayed hyperenhancement in

---

J.D. Schroeder, MD (✉)
Department of Radiology, University of Colorado,
Adjoint Associate Professor, Aurora, CO, USA
e-mail: joyce.schroeder@stanfordalumni.org

B. Fenster, MD, FACC, FACP, FASE
Division of Cardiology, Department of Medicine, National Jewish Health,
1400 Jackson St., Denver, CO 80206, USA
e-mail: fensterb@njhealth.org

the myocardium is not a specific sign for cardiac sarcoidosis, the MRI findings can be used as a complement to other imaging modalities and clinical and laboratory data in the diagnostic evaluation process. In a study of 81 patients with sarcoidosis, Patel et al. reported that delayed enhancement cardiac MRI is more than twice as sensitive for cardiac involvement as current (2009) consensus criteria [1]. In a study of 155 patients with systemic sarcoidosis, Greulich et al. report the presence of myocardial scar indicated by late gadolinium enhancement was the best independent predictor of potentially lethal events, yielding a Cox hazard ratio of 31.6 [2].

In addition to the use of DHE sequences for the detection of scar, typical Cardiac MRI protocols provide whole heart evaluation including cardiac anatomy, wall motion, function and perfusion as well as the evaluation of the mediastinum, hila and lungs for extra-cardiac signs of sarcoidosis. Cardiac MRI provides substantial advantages over other imaging modalities in the evaluation of the heart, including multi-sequence evaluation without ionizing radiation, higher spatial resolution than myocardial SPECT imaging, and greater tissue characterization than computed tomography (CT) or echocardiogram. In addition to diagnosis of disease, DHE imaging may also be useful for assessment of response to steroid therapy.

Although Cardiac MRI exams have typically been relatively long in duration for the patient (up to an hour), with the advent of streamlined MRI protocols, faster MRI hardware and a larger base of experienced MRI Technologists, Cardiac MRI exams are increasingly becoming a routine part of imaging department workflows.

Cardiac MRI Techniques

A typical Cardiac MRI protocol for the evaluation of cardiac sarcoidosis uses multiple sequences [3–5], as illustrated in Fig. 5.1. Scout images are performed to orient the imaging planes. Dark blood, T2 weighted and inversion recovery sequences are performed to assess anatomy and to assess the myocardium for evidence of high signal intensity edema or inflammation. Cinematic (cine), or movie, ECG-gated sequences generate time-resolved imaging of cardiac motion in the short axis (SA), horizontal long axis (HLA) and vertical long axis (VLA) planes. Cine three-chamber sequences demonstrate left ventricular (LV) inflow and outflow. After the administration of gadolinium-based intravenous contrast, dynamic perfusion images are acquired to assess for myocardial perfusion defects or scar. Perfusion images are often acquired in two planes, SA and HLA. Post-contrast axial images are acquired through the chest for evaluation of the mediastinum, hila and lungs.

5 Diagnosis II: Imaging of Cardiac Sarcoidosis with Cardiac MRI, PET and SPECT

The technique of delayed hyperenhancement (DHE) imaging uses an initial T1 scout sequence for determination of the correct inversion time in order to produce nulling (or dark signal intensity) of the myocardium. The correct inversion time is selected by the MR technologist or physician visually inspecting the T1 scout images; the inversion time is selected that shows uniform dark signal intensity within the myocardium. This inversion time is used for subsequent delayed images, typically acquired at 10–15 min after the intravenous contrast injection for the left ventricle. DHE images are usually acquired in three planes: SA, HLA and VLA. DHE imaging can also be targeted for the right ventricle, typically acquired 8–10 min after the intravenous contrast injection.

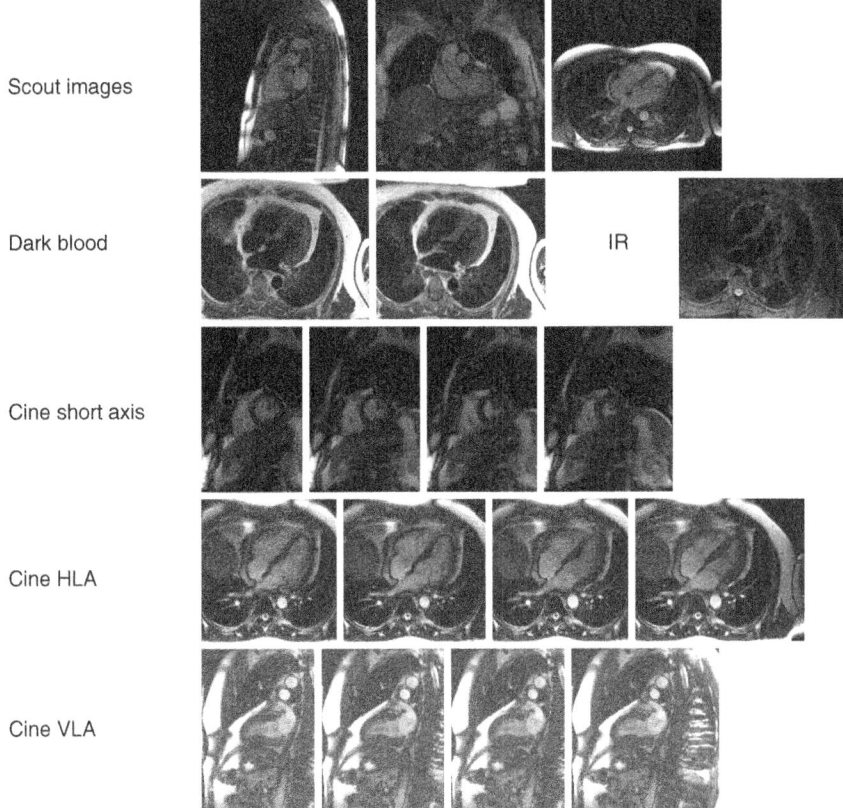

Fig. 5.1 Typical cardiac MRI protocol/sequences for imaging for cardiac sarcoidosis, including: scout images; dark blood; T2 weighted; inversion recovery; cinematic (cine) short axis (SA), horizontal long axis (HLA), and vertical long axis (VLA); three chamber; post-gadolinium intravenous contrast perfusion, axial chest, T1 scout and delayed hyperenhancement in SA, HLA and VLA planes. Post-processing is performed at either the MR console or on an independent workstation

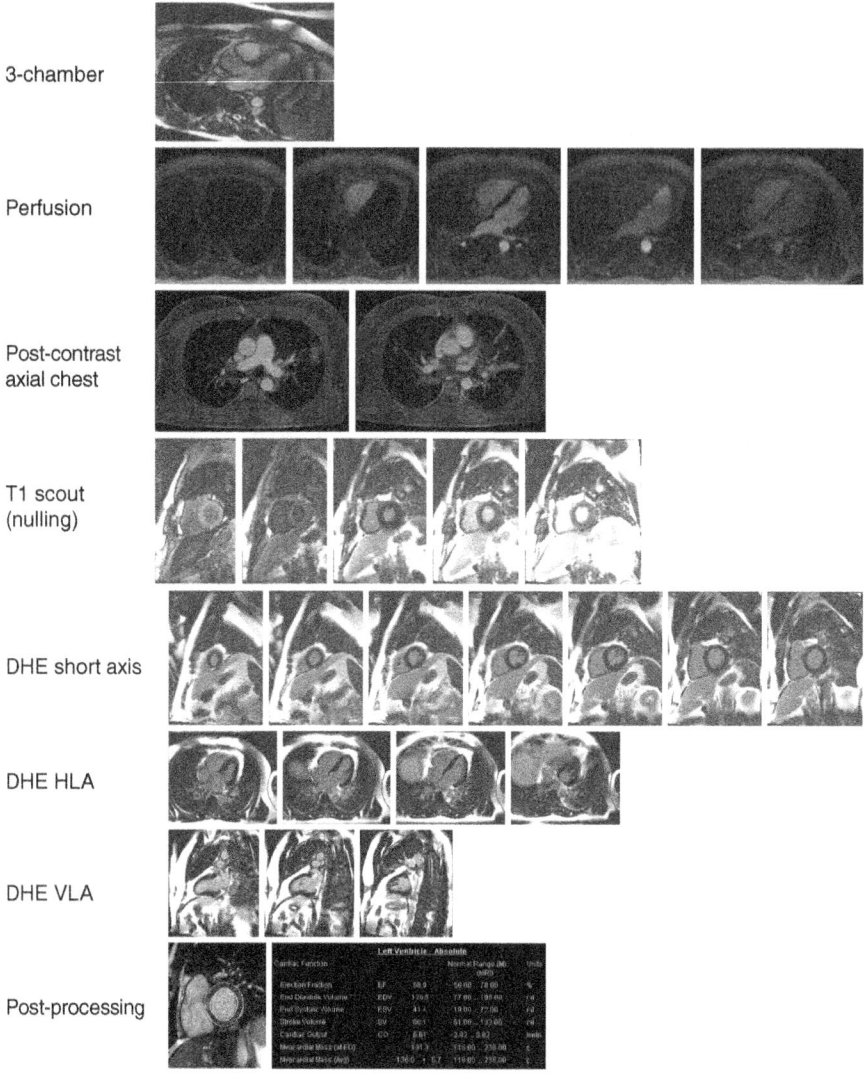

Fig. 5.1 (continued)

Post-processing of Cardiac MRI images, performed either at the MRI console or on an independent workstation, generates quantitative measures including ejection fraction, end diastolic/systolic volumes, stroke volume, cardiac output and myocardial mass [6].

Cardiac MRI exams are performed on either 1.5 or 3.0 Tesla magnetic resonance scanners. A flat set of receiver coils placed on the patient's chest during the exam contains parallel coils to improve signal-to-noise ratio and decrease exam acquisition time.

Cardiac MRI Imaging Features

Imaging Features and Patterns of Disease

Post-inflammatory Scarring

Cardiac sarcoidosis is characterized by patchy foci of high signal intensity in the myocardium on DHE imaging (Fig. 5.2). Foci of hyperenhancement are often located in basal or subepicardial regions but can be seen throughout the LV or RV myocardium [7]. Single foci of DHE may be subtle (Figs. 5.3 and 5.4), necessitating careful attention to MRI technique and consideration of artifacts.

Acute Inflammation

The inflammatory phase is characterized by focal wall thickening due to infiltration or edema, wall motion abnormalities and high T2 signal intensity [8]. Pathologic features of cardiac sarcoidosis include patchy infiltration of the myocardium in successive stages: edema, non-caseating granulomas, and finally fibrosis or scar [9]. T2 weighted imaging is increasingly being used for tissue characterization in acute myocardial processes.

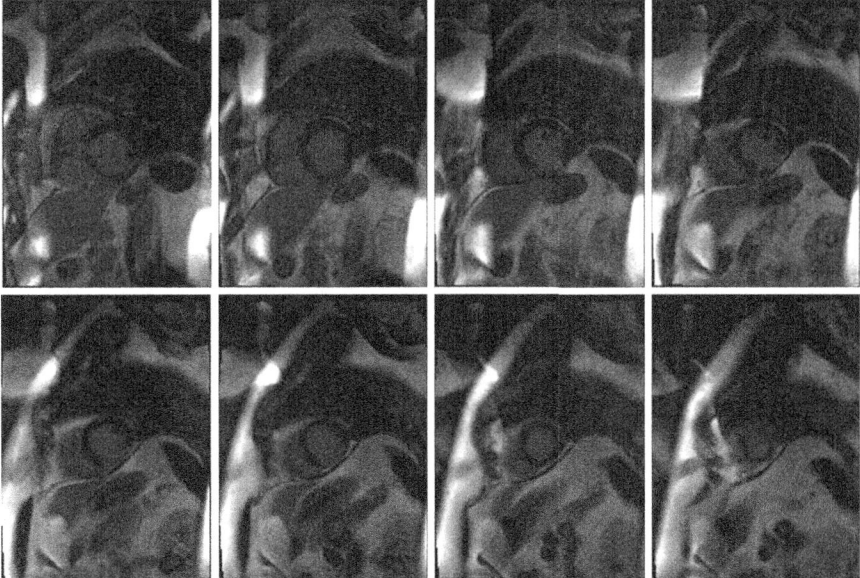

Fig. 5.2 62 year old man with a history of sarcoidosis and non-sustained ventricular tachycardia on Holter monitor. Short axis DHE images show patchy delayed hyperenhancement in the mid inferior and lateral left ventricular walls

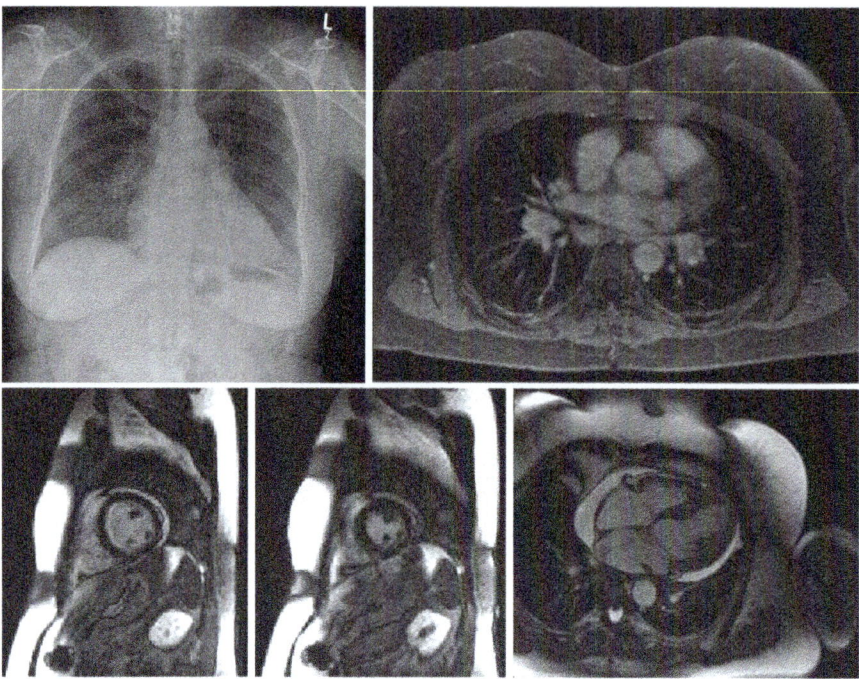

Fig. 5.3 48 year old woman with a history of opthalmic sarcoidosis. Chest radiograph and axial post-contrast MRI images show right hilar lymphadenopathy. Short axis and horizontal long axis DHE images show mild patchy delayed hyperenhancement in the inferolateral left ventricular wall and a small pericardial effusion

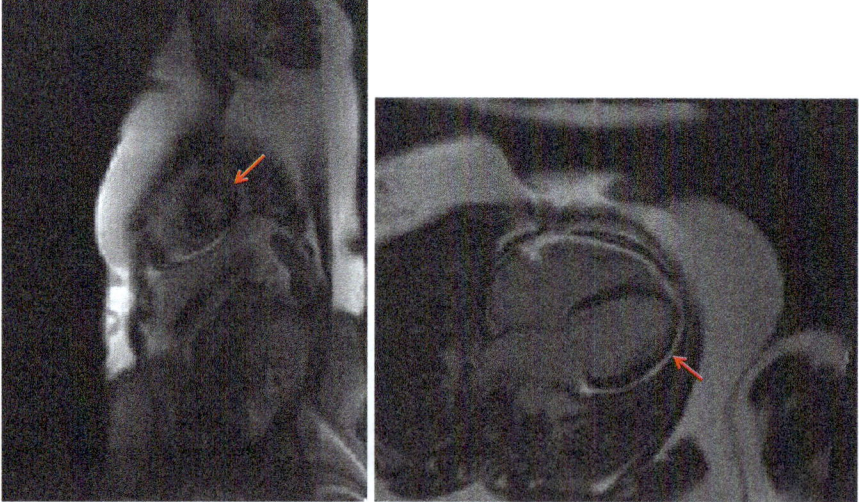

Fig. 5.4 61 year old woman with a history of sarcoidosis with mediastinal and abdominal lymphadenopathy, inducible ventricular tachycardia/ventricular fibrillation and frequent PVCs. Short axis and horizontal long axis DHE images show mild focal delayed hyperenhancement in the apical lateral wall (*arrows*). The patient subsequently received an implantable cardioverter defibrillator (ICD)

Wall Motion Abnormality

Three-plane (SA, HLA and VLA) cine imaging is used to assess wall motion. On visual analysis, hypokinetic, akinetic or dyskinetic foci of wall motion abnormality can be secondary to scarred or inflamed myocardium. Navigator tools can be used to confirm wall motion abnormalities in multiple planes.

Associated Features

Depending on the location and extent of cardiac involvement by sarcoidosis, associated features may include ventricular aneurysm or valvular involvement. The pericardium may become thickening and involved by sarcoidosis. Pericardial effusion is not uncommon. Extensive cardiac involvement by sarcoidosis may lead to congestive heart failure. Pulmonary hypertension is common in sarcoidosis (see Chap. 13) with imaging features including central pulmonary enlargement, right heart enlargement and possibly severe pulmonary parenchymal disease including nodularity, architectural distortion and fibrosis.

Differential Diagnosis for Myocardial DHE

Patchy delayed hyperenhancement in the myocardium is not a specific sign for cardiac sarcoidosis. Delayed hyperenhancement can be seen in infarction and other myocardial processes that cause myocardial necrosis, infiltration or fibrosis, including myocarditis, hypertrophic cardiomyopathy, amyloidosis, sarcoidosis and other myocardial conditions [10]. When DHE is in a coronary artery vascular distribution and not mid-myocardial in location, the differential diagnosis includes ischemia/infarct (Fig. 5.5).

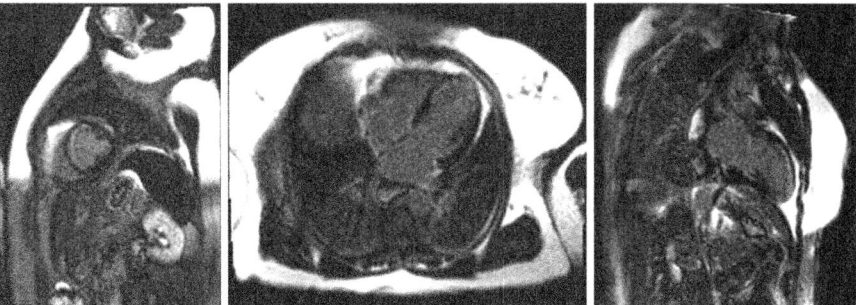

Fig. 5.5 57 year old woman with a history of left anterior descending (LAD) coronary artery disease with myocardial infarction. Multiplanar DHE images show delayed hyperenhancement in the LAD vascular territory

Extracardiac Findings of Sarcoidosis

Sarcoidosis can involve multiple anatomic structures typically within the field-of-view of a Cardiac MRI or PET/CT exam, including the pericardium, mediastinal and hilar lymph nodes, axillary lymph nodes, the lungs, upper abdominal lymph nodes, spleen, retroperitoneal lymph nodes and bones. Features of pulmonary sarcoidosis include mediastinal and hilar lymphadenopathy, nodularity, centrilobular nodularity, reticular abnormality, ground glass attenuation, perihilar confluent opacities, architectural distortion and pulmonary fibrosis. [^{18}F]fluorodeoxyglucose (FDG) positron emission tomography (PET) whole body imaging can be used for staging, identification of occult sites of disease and identification of sites suitable for biopsy [11].

Limitations of Cardiac MRI in the Diagnosis of Cardiac Sarcoidosis

Cardiac MRI is not a specific imaging modality for cardiac sarcoidosis and attention to correct MRI protocols and technique as well as artifacts and differential considerations is important. Limitations for Cardiac MRI include the length of the scan for the patient (up to an hour) and the geometry of the MRI scanner. Patients with claustrophobia may not be able to tolerate the exam length or proximity of the circular magnet bore and flat chest coils. Patient size may be an issue as obese patients may not fit into the typical 60 cm magnet bore depending on distribution of body adiposity, although 70 cm MRI scanner bores are increasingly available. Contraindications to an MRI exam include renal impairment (estimated glomerular filtration rate less than 30 mL/kg/min) due to the risk of gadolinium-induced nephrogenic systemic fibrosis. The presence of metallic fragments or any non-MRI-compliant materials within the body including conventional pacemakers are contraindications to MRI.

MR-compatible pacemakers are now available and acceptable cardiac MRI image quality is possible without substantial image degradation due to artifacts (Fig. 5.6). MR-conditional pacemakers may make the benefits of cardiac MRI imaging more available for patients with pacemakers [12], both in the diagnosis and followup of cardiac disease.

PET/CT for the Evaluation of Cardiac Sarcoidosis

PET/CT is used in the evaluation for cardiac sarcoidosis by assessing for hypermetabolic activity within the myocardium, implying inflammation, using a PET protocol designed to suppress normal myocardial glucose uptake.

5 Diagnosis II: Imaging of Cardiac Sarcoidosis with Cardiac MRI, PET and SPECT

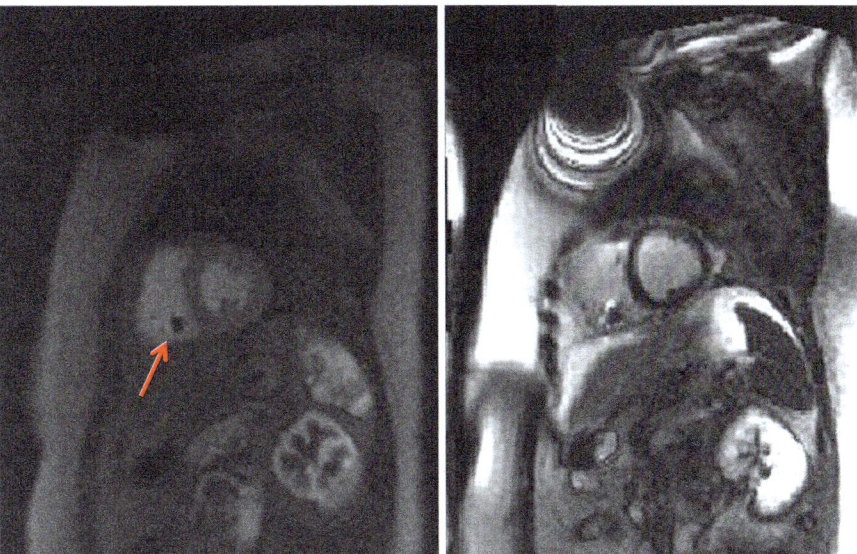

Fig. 5.6 37 year old woman with a history of atrial tachycardia ablation. Short axis perfusion and DHE images show MR-compatible pacemaker (Medtronic Advisa MRI SureScan) lead at the RV apex. Note artifact from the pacemaker device in soft tissues of the anterior upper chest wall. *Arrow* points to the pacemaker lead

Pre-exam patient instructions for a cardiac PET/CT exam include a low-to-no carbohydrate diet for 24 h and a total fast (except for water) for 6 h prior to the exam. The blood glucose target level is below 120 mG/dL. The radiopharmaceutical [^{18}F]fluorodeoxyglucose (FDG), dose range 10–12 mCi, is administered intravenously. After an incubation phase of 45–60 min the patient is scanned with CT and a 10 min 1-bed PET acquisition through the chest centered on the heart.

PET images and CT images are fused, or spatially registered, for review. The manifestations of cardiac sarcoidosis on PET/CT imaging may include patchy hypermetabolic activity in the myocardium (Fig. 5.7) or diffuse hypermetabolic activity in the left and/or right ventricular myocardium (Figs. 5.8 and 5.9). Patchy hypermetabolic activity may be due to inflammation. Diffuse myocardial hypermetabolic activity may be due to inflammation or, alternatively, due to failure to suppress the normal FDG-avid activity in the myocardium [13]. The relationship between PET findings in cardiac sarcoidosis and clinical outcomes is not well known. Blankstein et al. report that the presence of focal perfusion defects (assessed by rubidium-82) and FDG uptake on cardiac PET identifies patients at higher risk of death or ventricular tachycardia [14]. In a meta-analysis study of seven studies and 164 patients, Youssef et al. report a high diagnostic accuracy for ^{18}F-FDG PET (89 % sensitivity, 78 % specificity) although limitations include the small number of heterogeneous studies and small number of patients [15].

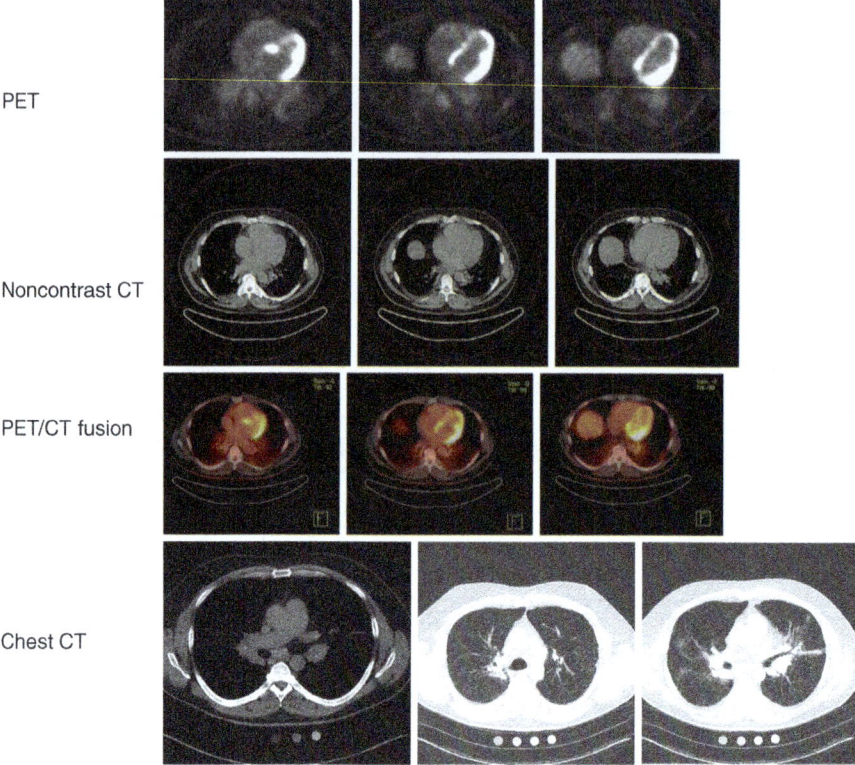

Fig. 5.7 42 year old man with a history of sarcoidosis. PET and PET/CT fusion images show patchy hypermetabolic activity in the left ventricular myocardium. Chest CT images show typical manifestations of pulmonary sarcoidosis including mediastinal and hilar lymphadenopathy, perihilar confluent masses with architectural distortion, and peribronchovascular nodularity

Hypermetabolic activity on PET/CT images secondary to sarcoidosis can also be seen in the pericardium and mediastinal and hilar lymphadenopathy.

As an extension of PET/CT techniques, hybrid PET-MR scanners are a new imaging modality for potential evaluation of cardiac sarcoidosis [16, 17].

Nuclear Medicine Myocardial SPECT Imaging for the Evaluation of Cardiac Sarcoidosis

Nuclear medicine technetium (99mTc) sestamibi myocardial single-photon emission computed tomography (SPECT) imaging for the assessment of cardiac sarcoidosis uses a standard cardiac SPECT protocol. A "reverse perfusion defect" refers to

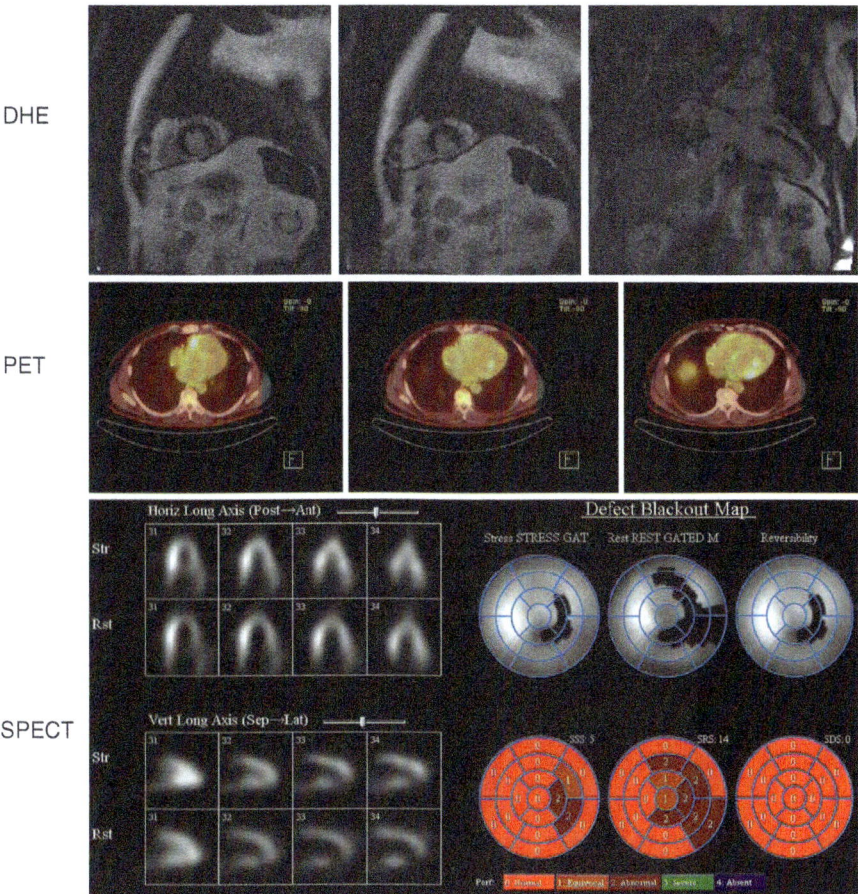

Fig. 5.8 61 year old man with a history of sarcoidosis diagnosed on pericardial biopsy. Short axis and vertical long axis DHE images show delayed hyperenhancement in the inferior wall that may be secondary to known coronary artery disease and previous infarct. DHE was also present in the basal septum. PET images show patchy hypermetabolic activity in the RV free wall, interventricular septum, and lateral LV wall. An implantable cardioverter defibrillator (ICD) is present. Nuclear medicine myocardial (SPECT) scan shows scarring in the inferolateral wall and additional perfusion abnormalities at rest consistent with reverse distribution that may be manifestation of myocardial sarcoidosis

perfusion abnormalities seen on rest imaging that are not present or less prominent on stress imaging. Myocardial perfusion abnormalities in sarcoidosis are reversible after pharmacological dilation which may be due to possible microvascular constriction in myocardial sarcoidosis; this phenomenon is referred to as "reverse distribution" but is not specific for cardiac sarcoidosis [18]. See Figs. 5.8 and 5.9. Delayed hyperenhancement has been shown to be associated with reduction of regional wall motion and thallium perfusion defects [19, 20].

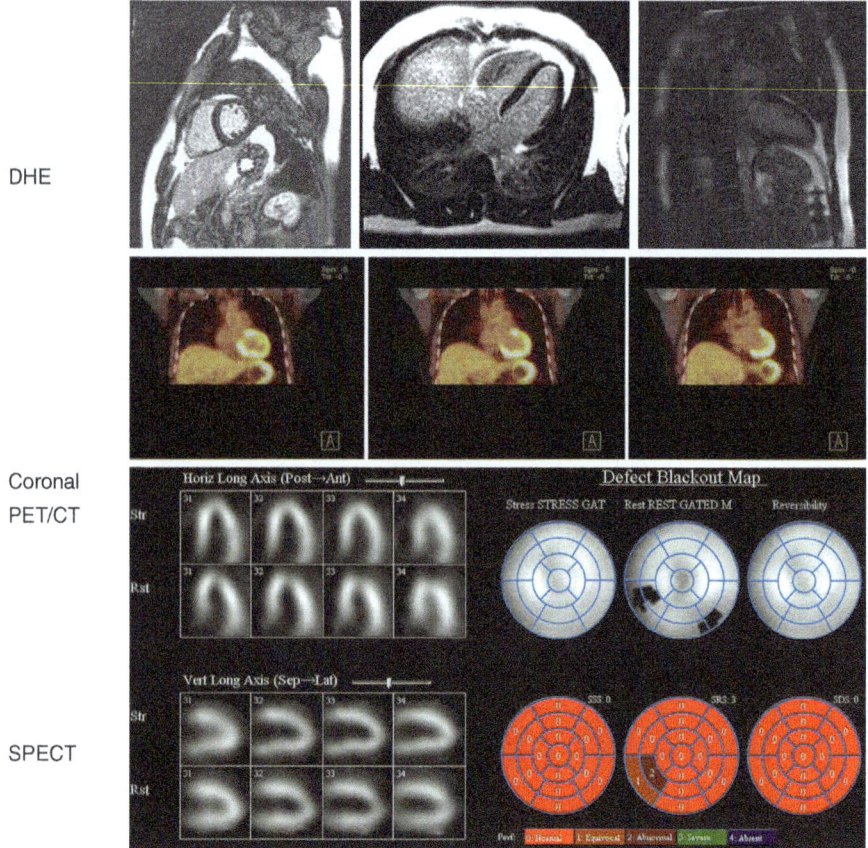

Fig. 5.9 36 year old man with a history of sarcoidosis including lymphadenopathy, liver, cardiac and gastric involvement. History of first degree AV block, palpitations and inducible ventricular tachycardia on electrophysiology (EP) study. DHE images show mild diffuse mid-myocardial delayed hyperenhancement, possibly artifactual but confirmed on multiplanar images. Coronal PET/CT fusion images show diffuse LV hypermetabolic activity. Nuclear medicine myocardial (SPECT) scan shows perfusion abnormalities at rest, possible manifestation of myocardial sarcoidosis

Correlation Between Imaging Modalities

Cardiac MRI, cardiac PET/CT and nuclear medicine myocardial SPECT imaging are all non-specific imaging modalities for cardiac sarcoidosis. However, the interpretation of these imaging studies in the context of the clinical history and other laboratory results, imaging and biopsy findings can be useful in the diagnosis of cardiac sarcoidosis. More on the multimodality approach to imaging cardiac sarcoidosis will be discussed in Chap. 7.

Freeman et al. describe a scoring system using common clinical tests to predict positive imaging findings using Cardiac MRI or FDG-cardiac PET and report that scoring system positivity was driven more by Cardiac MRI than FDG-cardiac PET [21].

Conclusion

Imaging of cardiac sarcoidosis with Cardiac MRI, PET and SPECT provides a rich set of tools for the evaluation of myocardial scar, edema, inflammation, functional abnormalities and associated features. However, these imaging modalities are not individually specific for cardiac sarcoidosis and the role of imaging in the diagnosis and followup of cardiac sarcoidosis requires careful integration with laboratory and clinical data.

Pearls of Wisdom
1. Cardiac MRI, PET and SPECT imaging modalities are not individually specific for cardiac sarcoidosis and the role of imaging in the diagnosis and followup of cardiac sarcoidosis requires careful integration with laboratory and clinical data.
2. Cardiac magnetic resonance imaging (MRI) is a useful tool in the diagnosis of cardiac sarcoidosis primarily through the use of delayed hyperenhancement (DHE) sequences for the detection of bright (high signal intensity) scar in the myocardium; careful attention to MR technique and an understanding of artifacts is required.
3. PET/CT is used in the evaluation for cardiac sarcoidosis by assessing for hypermetabolic activity within the myocardium using a specialized protocol, however, myocardial hypermetabolic activity may be due to inflammation or, alternatively, failure to suppress the normal FDG-activity in the myocardium.

References

1. Patel MR, Cawley PJ, Heitner JF, et al. Detection of myocardial damage in patients with sarcoidosis. Circulation. 2009;120:1969–77.
2. Greulich S, Deluigi CC, Gloekler S, et al. CMR imaging predicts death and other adverse events in suspected cardiac sarcoidosis. J Am Coll Cardiol Img. 2013;6:501–11.
3. O'Donnell DH, Abbara S, Chaithiraphan V, et al. Cardiac MR imaging of nonischemic cardiomyopathies: imaging protocols and spectra of appearances. Radiology. 2012;262(2):403–22.
4. Parsai C, O'Hanlon R, Prasad SK, et al. Diagnostic and prognostic value of cardiovascular magnetic resonance in non-ischaemic cardiomyopathies. J Cardiovasc Magn Reson. 2012;12:54.
5. Kramer CM, Barkhausen J, Flamm SD, et al. Standardized cardiovascular magnetic resonance imaging (CMR) protocols, society for cardiovascular magnetic resonance: board of trustees task force on standardized protocols. J Cardiovasc Magn Reson. 2008;10:35.
6. Schulz-Menger J, Bluemke DA, Bremerich J, et al. Standardized image interpretation and post processing in cardiovascular magnetic resonance: society for cardiovascular magnetic resonance (SCMR) board of trustees task force on standardized post processing. J Cardiovasc Magn Reson. 2013;15:35.
7. Ichinose A, Otani H, Oikawa M, et al. MRI of cardiac sarcoidosis: basal and subepicardial localization of myocardial lesions and their effect on left ventricular function. AJR. 2008;191:862–9.
8. Schatka I, Bengel FM. Advanced imaging of cardiac sarcoidosis. J Nucl Med. 2014;55:99–106.

9. Mirakhur A, Anca N, Mikami Y, et al. T2-weighted imaging of the heart—a pictorial review. Eur J Radiol. 2013;82:1755–62.
10. Ordovas KG, Higgins CB. Delayed contrast enhancement on MR images of myocardium: past, present, future. Radiology. 2011;261(2):358–74.
11. Sobic-Saranovic D, Artiko V, Obradovic V. FDG PET imaging in sarcoidosis. Semin Nucl Med. 2013;43:404–11.
12. Bhandiwad AR, et al. Cardiovascular magnetic resonance with an MR compatible pacemaker. J Cardiovasc Magn Reson. 2013;15:18.
13. Maurer AH, Burshteyn M, Adler LP, et al. How to differentiate benign versus malignant cardiac and paracardiac ^{18}F FDG uptake at oncologic PET/CT. RadioGraphics. 2011;31: 1287–305.
14. Blankstein R, Osborne M, Naya M, et al. Cardiac positron emission tomography enhances prognostic assessments of patients with suspected cardiac sarcoidosis. J Am Coll Cardiol. 2014;63:329–36.
15. Youssef G, Leung E, Mylonas I, et al. The use of ^{18}F-FDG in the diagnosis of cardiac sarcoidosis: a systematic review and metaanalysis including the Ontario experience. J Nucl Med. 2012;53:241–8.
16. O'Meara C, Menezes LJ, White SK, et al. Initial experience of imaging cardiac sarcoidosis using hybrid PET-MR—a technologist's case study. J Cardiovasc Magn Reson. 2013;15 Suppl 1:T1.
17. Torigian DA, Zaidi H, Kwee TC, et al. PET/MR imaging: technical aspects and potential clinical applications. Radiology. 2013;267:26–44.
18. Sekhri V, Sanal S, DeLorinzo LJ, et al. Cardiac sarcoidosis: a comprehensive review. Arch Med Sci. 2011;7(4):546–54.
19. Tadamura E, Yamamuro M, Kubo S, et al. Effectiveness of delayed enhanced MRI for identification of cardiac sarcoidosis: comparison with radionuclide imaging. AJR. 2005;185: 110–1.
20. Vignaux O. Cardiac sarcoidosis: spectrum of MRI features. AJR. 2005;184:249–54.
21. Freeman AM, Curran-Everett D, Weinberger HD, et al. Predictors of cardiac sarcoidosis using commonly available cardiac studies. Am J Cardiol. 2013;112:280–5.

Chapter 6
Nuclear Imaging (SPECT and PET) in Cardiac Sarcoidosis

Ron Blankstein and Sharmila Dorbala

Abstract Nuclear imaging techniques are increasingly used for evaluating patients with known or suspected cardiac sarcoidosis. In addition to assessing the likelihood that cardiac sarcoidosis is present or absent, data from these tests can also be used to risk stratify patients, and thus inform the potential need for various therapies. The most commonly used techniques include resting myocardial perfusion imaging (MPI), which can be performed with either single photon emission computed tomography (SPECT) or positron emission tomography (PET), and imaging for myocardial inflammation using F18-Flurodeoxyglucose (FDG). Patients who have significant myocardial inflammation – as detected by FDG uptake – should be considered for anti-inflammatory therapies, although data regarding the benefit of such treatment remains limited. Among patients who are treated with anti-inflammatory therapies, serial PET exams may be useful for determining the response to therapy. The development of future tracers will further increase the capabilities of nuclear imaging techniques to guide the diagnosis and treatment of patients with cardiac sarcoidosis.

Introduction

Nuclear imaging techniques offer a unique ability to evaluate patients with known or suspected cardiac sarcoidosis. The most commonly used techniques include resting myocardial perfusion imaging (MPI), which can be performed with either single photon emission computed tomography (SPECT) or positron emission tomography (PET), and imaging for myocardial inflammation using F18-Flurodeoxyglucose (FDG). This chapter will describe how these techniques, including older methods such as Gallium-67 imaging, are performed and used in evaluating patients with known or suspected cardiac sarcoidosis. We will then provide an overview of potential future tracers which are currently being investigated.

R. Blankstein, MD, FACC (✉) • S. Dorbala, MD, MPH
Non-invasive Cardiovascular Imaging Program, Department of Medicine (Cardiovascular Division) and Department of Radiology, Brigham and Women's Hospital,
Harvard Medical School, Shapiro Room 5096, 75 Francis Street, Boston, MA 02115, USA
e-mail: rblankstein@partners.org; sdorbala@partners.org

© Springer International Publishing Switzerland 2015
A.M. Freeman, H.D. Weinberger (eds.), *Cardiac Sarcoidosis:*
Key Concepts in Pathogenesis, Disease Management, and Interesting Cases,
DOI 10.1007/978-3-319-14624-9_6

Gallium-67 Imaging for Cardiac Sarcoidosis

Gallium-67, a SPECT radiotracer with a physical half-life of 78 h, has been used extensively for the evaluation of systemic and pulmonary sarcoidosis since the early 1970s with reported sensitivities of 60–90 %. Several studies have shown that Gallium-67 uptake by sarcoidosis granulomas may reflect increased capillary permeability or increased iron binding proteins such as transferrin or lactoferrin, which are increased at sites of inflammation [1]. Gallium-67 imaging is performed as planar imaging or SPECT, with intravenous injection of 150–220 MBq (4–6 mCi) followed by imaging 24–72 h later, using a medium energy parallel hole collimator, with three photopeaks (93, 184, 296 KeV) for 10 min [2]. When used for the evaluation of cardiac sarcoidosis, Gallium-67 imaging has typically been performed in conjunction with Thallium-201 myocardial perfusion imaging [3]. The sensitivity of Gallium-67 to detect cardiac sarcoidosis is low (estimated range 0–36 %) although the specificity approaches 100 % [4]. Reflecting the poor sensitivity of this technique, in one small study of patients with positive F-18 FDG uptake by PET, only 23 % showed abnormal Gallium uptake in the heart [5]. Improvement in myocardial perfusion and reduction in Gallium-67 uptake have been described after successful therapy for sarcoidosis [3, 6]. However, due to limited image quality, low sensitivity and the greater availability of PET technology for imaging F-18 FDG, Gallium-67 imaging is currently not used widely in clinical practice for the diagnosis of cardiac sarcoidosis.

Rest Myocardial Perfusion Imaging

Resting myocardial perfusion imaging (MPI) can be performed using either SPECT or PET techniques (Table 6.1). While PET imaging offers superior image quality, improved spatial resolution, and robust attenuation correction, this technique is less widely available. The currently available PET radiotracers include rubidium-82 (which requires an onsite generator) and N-13 ammonia (which requires a cyclotron for production). Alternatively SPECT MPI can be performed with either thallium-201 or technetium-99m. Due to improved image quality and a lower radiation dose, the use of technetium-99m is preferred for SPECT imaging. In addition, when available the use of attenuation correction is strongly suggested.

While the use of rest MPI is extremely helpful when interpreting FDG PET images, the value of rest MPI alone imaging is limited. For instance, in early stages of cardiac sarcoidosis, the rest MPI can be completely normal. Among patients with suspected cardiac sarcoidosis, the presence of a resting perfusion defect is often non-specific as the differential diagnosis for this finding includes: (a) scar and/or inflammation from cardiac sarcoidosis; (b) artifact, such as an attenuation artifact; (c) scar from prior myocardial infarction; or (d) hibernating myocardium.

Table 6.1 Data provided by nuclear imaging techniques

Variable	Technique	What it means in cardiac sarcoidosis?
Resting myocardial perfusion imaging	Can be performed by either SPECT or PET myocardial perfusion imaging	Resting perfusion defects can be due to either scar and/or intense inflammation causing compression of the microvasculature
Imaging inflammation with F18 flurodeoxyglucose	Performed with PET	Following adequate patient preparation (see text), increased FDG uptake represents myocardial inflammation
	Can be quantified	
	May improve upon treatment with systemic anti-inflammatory medications	
	Can be used to visualize areas of increased FDG uptake outside the heart	Requires suppression of glucose uptake by normal myocardium and exclusion of other causes of increased FDG uptake by the myocardium

Inflammation Imaging Using F18-Flurodeoxyglucose

F18-FDG is used to image myocardial inflammation based on the fact that inflammatory cells such as macrophages have a higher metabolic activity. After crossing the cell membrane, F18-becomes phosphorylated by the enzyme hexokinase and then becomes trapped inside the cells, thus allowing for imaging. However, it is important to remember that FDG uptake by the myocardium is not specific to cardiac sarcoidosis, and must be interpreted in the context of the patient's medical history as well as the dietary conditions that were employed at the time of image acquisition. For instance, patients with coronary heart disease who have hibernating myocardium (i.e. reduced perfusion due to chronic ischemia accompanied by a shift in metabolic pathways to favor glucose uptake instead of free fatty acids) may have FDG uptake. Other inflammatory myopathies, such as active myocarditis or systemic rheumatological conditions with cardiac involvement may also be associated with increased FDG uptake by the myocardium. Finally, FDG uptake by the myocardium – especially when diffuse or confined to the lateral wall – may be a normal variant, particularly when imaging is performed in the non-fasted state and/or under states of high insulin.

The Logistics of Performing FDG PET Imaging

Patient Preparation

Adequate patient preparation to suppress the physiologic uptake of FDG by the normal myocardium is essential when performing PET imaging for inflammation. There are multiple protocols (Table 6.2) that have been used by different centers and no clear data to support the superiority of any one particular method. Cheng et al. studied 63 patients referred for oncologic imaging, and found that a low carbohydrate diet

Table 6.2 Methods used to suppress FDG from the normal myocardium

Protocol	Comments/tips
High fat low carbohydrate diet × 2 meals followed by fast of at least 4 h	Good experience by our group; used in Blankstein et al. [9]
High fat low carbohydrate (HFLC) diet + prolonged fast	Supported by Demeure et al. [8]
Low carbohydrate (LC) diet followed by fast	Supported by Cheng et al. [7]
Prolonged fast	Suggest at least 18 h fast
	Supported by Morooka et al. [15]
High fat low carbohydrate diet supplemented by high fat beverage 1 h prior to FDG injection	Inferior to HFLC diet or LC diet followed by fast [7, 8]
Heparin administration	Dose 50 IU/kg used in some studies, but lower doses may also be effective (avoid administering in dextrose); inferior to long term fasting [15]

followed by a fast resulted in greater reduction in SUV (versus a controlled group of patients following an unrestricted diet) than a high fat low carbohydrate diet in which patients also drank a 250 cc beverage of mostly non-saturated fat 1 h prior to FDG injection [7]. Recently, Demeure et al. showed that a high fat low carbohydrate diet followed by a 12 h fast effectively suppressed FDG uptake in most (8 out 9) subjects. In their study, and consistent with the results of Cheng et al. administering an extra fat load 1 h before the scan did not offer any benefit [8]. Based on these two studies, administering a high fat beverage prior to imaging is not recommended. It is possible that such an approach of overloading the myocardium with free fatty acids could increase myocardial oxygen consumption leading to a paradoxical increase in glucose metabolism. In general, even under optimal conditions, approximately 10 % of patients may have diffuse non-specific uptake of FDG by the myocardium.

At our center we recommend a high fat/low carbohydrate diet for two meals prior to the scan followed by a fast of at least 4 h. Prior to imaging, all patients are asked about their diet, and if there are any issues (i.e. patient inadvertently ate carbohydrates), the study is postponed. In addition, patients are asked to avoid any strenuous exercise for 1 day prior to the scan. In patients who are unable to follow this diet (e.g. NPO for other medical reasons) we suggest a prolonged fast of at least 18 h.

Imaging Protocol

FDG image acquisition is typically performed 90 min after the administration of 10–12 mCi of F18-FDG although a shorter uptake period of 60 min has also been used by some centers. Our suggested protocol includes:

1. Low dose CT images for attenuation correction
2. Whole body FDG imaging – imaging from cerebellum to thigh utilizing multiple bed acquisitions performed in 3D (approximately four to five bed acquisitions

are needed, depending on patient's height as well as z-axis coverage per bed position)
3. Cardiac FDG imaging – single bed 3D acquisition over the heart with longer acquisition duration (~10 min)

Whole body FDG is an important component of the cardiac PET exam as this information can identify the presence and severity of extra cardiac disease. When present, such disease may help inform the role of anti-inflammatory therapies. In addition, when the diagnosis of sarcoidosis is uncertain, the presence of extra cardiac FDG avid disease may identify potential biopsy targets that are more accessible than the heart. These images should be interpreted by a physician who is trained at body PET/CT as it is important to recognize normal distribution of FDG by various organs from pathologic uptake.

Image Interpretation

Image interpretation requires simultaneous visualization of both rest MPI and FDG PET images. Normal scans will have complete suppression of FDG from the myocardium with normal resting perfusion (Fig. 6.1). At times, patients without cardiac disease may also have diffuse homogenous uptake of FDG by the myocardium. This pattern should be distinguished from diffuse patchy myocardial involvement which can be seen in patients with extensive myocardial inflammation.

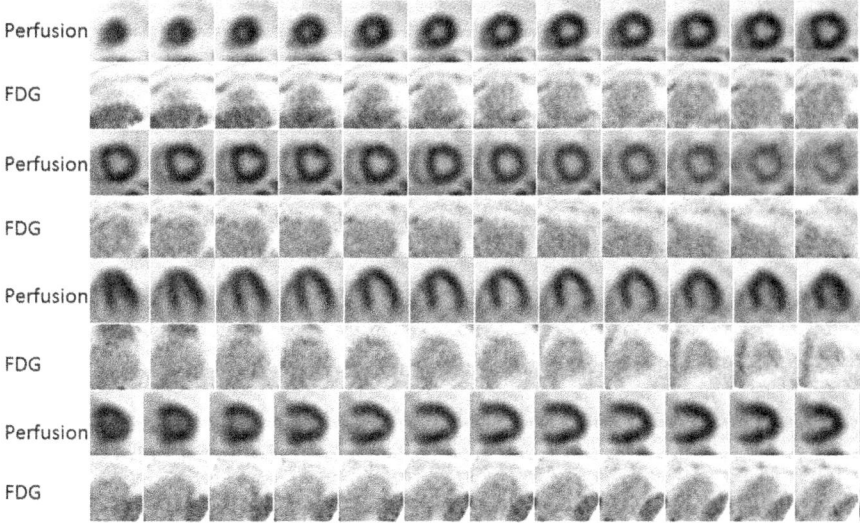

Fig. 6.1 Example of normal F-18 FDG PET/CT. Rest myocardial perfusion imaging demonstrates normal perfusion of the left ventricle with no defects. The cardiac FDG images show good suppression of FDG from the myocardium with no focal uptake involving the left or right ventricles

Most patients with cardiac involvement will exhibit a focal or focal-on-diffuse area of myocardial FDG uptake. Less frequently, focal areas of increased FDG uptake involving the right ventricle may also be seen, a finding which is associated with adverse prognosis [9].

In earlier stages of disease isolated FDG uptake may be seen without any perfusion defects. However, in more progressive stages of disease, resting perfusion defects may be present. While these defects are often due to the presence of scar, severe inflammation can also cause perfusion defects due to microvascular compression. Supporting this concept, we have observed that some patients can have a significant decrease in the size or intensity of resting perfusion defects following anti-inflammatory therapies. Patients with advanced "burnt out" disease will exhibit a large amount of scar with minimal or no FDG uptake.

One of the characteristic finding of cardiac PET in cardiac sarcoidosis is a perfusion/metabolism "mismatch" whereby areas of increased FDG also exhibit a resting perfusion defect (Fig. 6.2). However, it is noteworthy that such a mismatch pattern

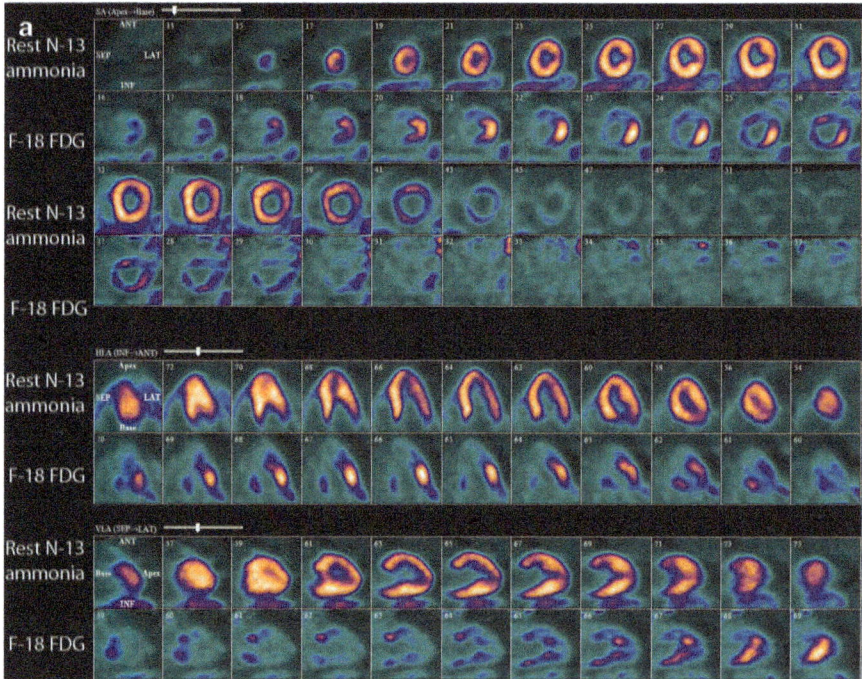

Fig. 6.2 Rest N-13 ammonia myocardial perfusion imaging and F-18 FDG PET/CT imaging (alternate rows) of a patient with biopsy proven cardiac sarcoidosis are shown at baseline (**a**) and after therapy (**b**). The images are displayed in standard cardiac projections of short axis (apex to base from left to right), horizontal long axis (inferior to anterior walls from left to right) and vertical long axis images (septum to lateral walls from left to right). The baseline study demonstrates a mild perfusion defect in the mid and basal anterolateral walls with a mismatch pattern (increased FDG uptake). The follow-up study demonstrates normal myocardial perfusion without perfusion defects and no myocardial FDG uptake (only blood pool activity is noted)

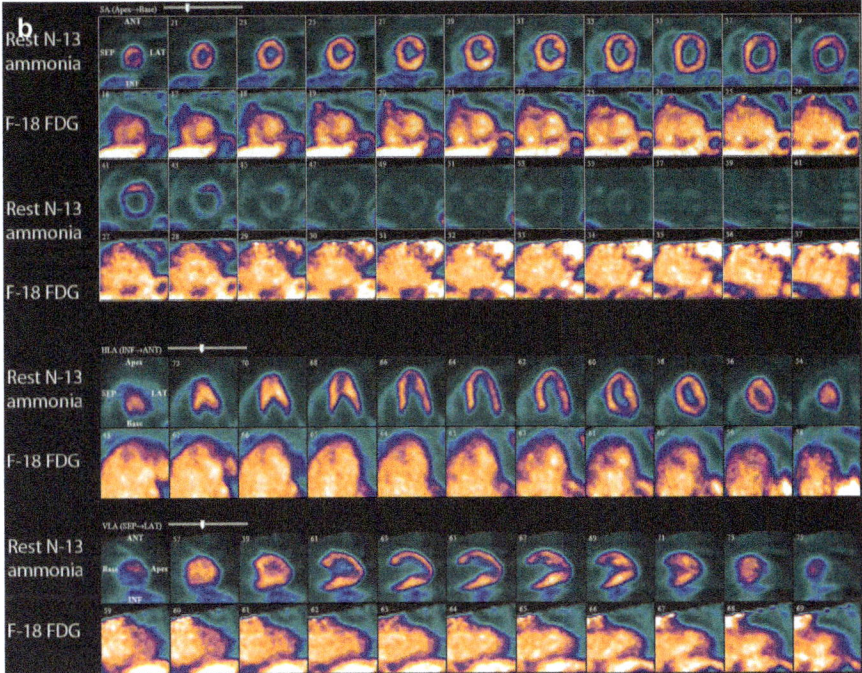

Fig. 6.2 (continued)

can also occur in patients with hibernating myocardium, and thus when the diagnosis of cardiac sarcoidosis is suspected based on such PET findings, it may be necessary to rule out the presence of obstructive coronary artery disease.

While Chap. 7 of this book has a more extensive discussion regarding the diagnostic and prognostic value of cardiac PET, it is important to note that abnormal PET findings are associated with a higher risk of ventricular tachycardia or death (Fig. 6.3). The risk of such events appears to be highest in patients who have abnormalities in both resting perfusion and FDG uptake [9].

Response to Therapy

A unique role of PET imaging with FDG is evaluating – both visually and quantitatively – how patients respond to immunosuppressive therapies. While some patients may have a significant response with complete resolution of inflammation (Figs. 6.2), other may demonstrate no significant change or even interval worsening. Since there is no data indicating the ideal drug, dose, or duration of therapy, and given the toxic side effect profiles of all anti-inflammatory agents, imaging may allow clinicians to select agents to which patients respond while limiting the duration of therapy and/or considering alternative agents when no significant

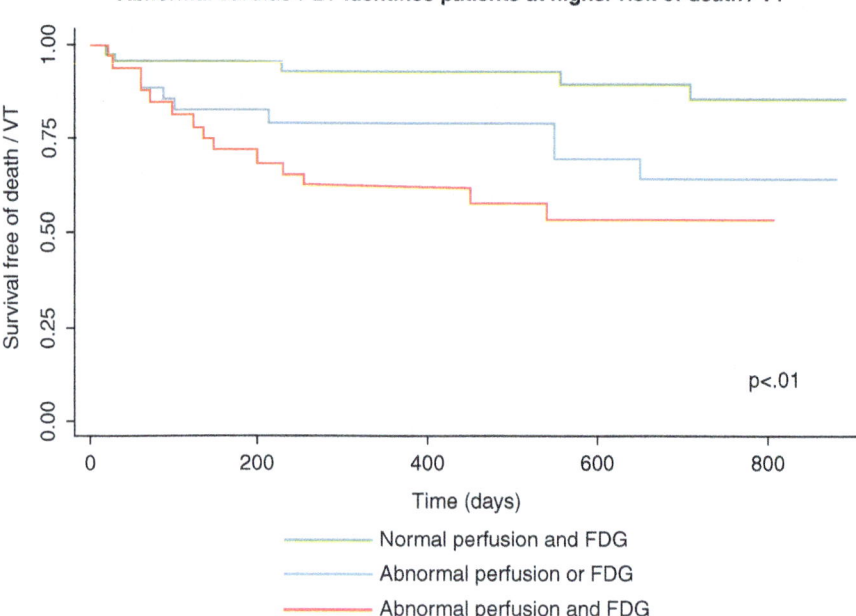

Fig. 6.3 Prognostic value of cardiac PET (With permission from Elsevier Publication. Source: Blankstein et al. [9])

benefit is observed. Further supporting the role of FDG imaging in following response to therapy, Osborne et al. have showed that among 23 patients who underwent serial PET exams during treatment for cardiac sarcoidosis, a reduction in the intensity (i.e. SUV max) or extent (i.e. volume of inflammation above a pre-specified SUV threshold) was associated with improvement in left ventricular ejection fraction.

However, it must be acknowledged that even when complete resolution of inflammation can be visualized by PET FDG, it is unknown if continuation of therapy at a lower dose has any role in preventing recurrence of disease. It is further unknown whether treatment is associated with a reduction in event rates, and if so, if this reduction is significant enough to warrant delaying or avoiding ICD therapy in patients who have inflammation prior to the development of significant scar or LV dysfunction.

There are multiple caveats that are important to keep in mind when comparing different imaging studies:

1. All studies should be performed in a similar fashion – same dietary preparation; same dose of injected activity; same time interval from FDG injection until image acquisition.
2. Whole body FDG images should be compared, as relying solely on the cardiac images may lead to errors from differences in normalization [10].

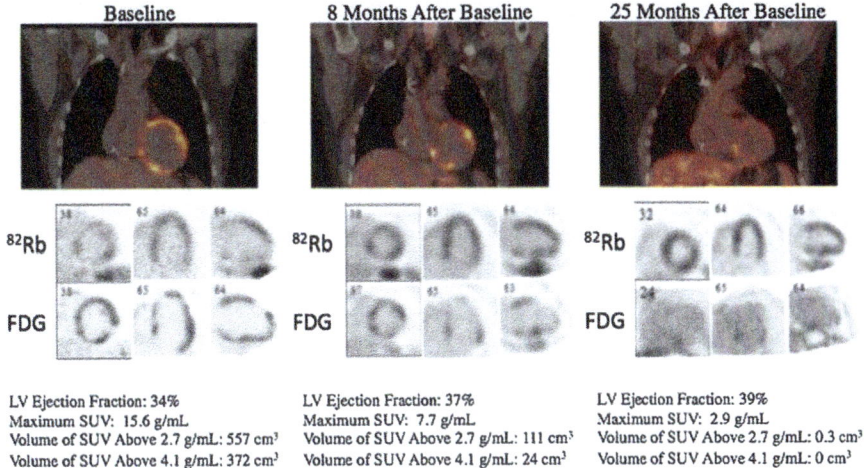

Fig. 6.4 Example of quantifying response to inflammation (Permission from Elsevier obtained by Ron Blankstein)

3. In addition to visual comparison, it is important to perform a quantitative comparison. This can be performed by comparing:

    (a) The intensity of inflammation – comparing SUV maximum value
    (b) The extent of inflammation – comparing the volume of myocardium that has FDG uptake above a pre-specified threshold.

    Figure 6.4 provides an example of using FDG imaging to assess the response to therapy.

Future Radiotracers for Imaging Cardiac Sarcoidosis

In addition to F-18 FDG and Gallium-67, several radiotracers are available to image inflammatory processes including Tc-99m or In -11 labeled white blood cells, Tc-99m labeled bisphosphonates, Tc-99m labeled nanocolloids and Tc-99m or In -11 labeled proteins, albumin, somatostatin receptor binding agents (Gallium-68 DOTA, Gallium-68 DOTANOC) [11]. In addition, Iodine-123-labeled 15-(p-iodophenyl)-3R,S-methylpentadecanoic acid (BMIPP), a fatty acid imaging agent has also been used in one small study of six patients with biopsy proven cardiac sarcoidosis along with Thallium-201 and shown to have a high specificity (100 %) and high negative predictive value (100 %) for the diagnosis of cardiac sarcoidosis [12]. There has been a growing interest in the use of Gallium-68, a PET radiotracer for imaging sarcoidosis. A clinical trial is now underway comparing Gallium Ga 68-DOTANOC, and gallium Ga 68-labeled DOTA with F-18 FDG PET [13]. In one recent study [14], 18 patients with biopsy proven systemic sarcoidosis (no myocardial sarcoidosis patients) were studied with Gallium-67 and 111

In-pentetreotide imaging. In this study, 111 In-pentetreotide imaging consistently showed better image quality. However, further studies are needed in order to better understand the role of this agent in evaluating patients with cardiac sarcoidosis [14].

In addition to developing better tracers for this disease, it will be important to develop more data relating to how SPECT and PET imaging results can be used to better risk stratify patients. Finally, standardized techniques will be needed in order to determine how to better quantify and follow disease activity, and whether this information can ultimately be used to enhance patient outcomes.

Pearls of Wisdom
1. Gallium-67 imaging for cardiac sarcoidosis is of limited value due to low sensitivity and is typically only used when F-18 FDG PET or cardiac MRI imaging are not available.
2. Increase uptake of Gallium-67 in the hilar nodes may be seen as a normal variant especially in smokers.

    - NOTE: Interested readers are referred to the procedure guideline document for other factors that may cause artifacts with Gallium-67 imaging. Reference: Seabold et al. [2]

3. When evaluating patients with known or suspected cardiac sarcoidosis, both rest MPI (with either SPECT or PET) and PET FDG imaging should be performed. Neither one alone is adequate for fully characterizing disease activity.
4. Prior to imaging myocardial FDG uptake, dietary preparation to reduce the uptake of FDG by the normal myocardium is essential. We suggest a high fat low carbohydrate diet for two meals followed by a fast of at least 4 h, although alternatively, this diet can also be followed by a prolonged fast. It is essential to provide patients with very specific instruction. On the day of testing, it is important to ensure that they were able to follow the diet before any imaging is performed.
5. Uptake of FDG by the lateral wall may represent a normal variant, particularly when (a) there is no perfusion defect involving the lateral wall; (b) the FDG uptake is homogenous (as opposed to patchy); and (c) the likelihood of cardiac disease is low.
6. Patients with advanced cardiac sarcoidosis may have "burnt out" disease with no (or little) FDG uptake. Such patients are more likely to have left ventricular systolic dysfunction. Patients with large amount of scar and reduced ejection fraction are less likely to have an improvement in ejection fraction following immunosuppressive therapy.
7. When interpreting FDG PET studies, it is essential to also acquire and interpret whole body FDG data in order to identify if there is any active extra cardiac disease. The presence of FDG avid disease outside the heart may also identify a site that is more amenable to biopsy than the heart.

References

1. Tzen KY, Oster ZH, Wagner Jr HN, Tsan MF. Role of iron-binding proteins and enhanced capillary permeability on the accumulation of gallium-67. J Nucl Med Off Publ Soc Nucl Med. 1980;21:31–5.
2. Seabold JE, et al. Procedure guideline for gallium scintigraphy in inflammation. Society of Nuclear Medicine. J Nucl Med Off Publ Soc Nucl Med. 1997;38:994–7.
3. Okayama K, et al. Diagnostic and prognostic value of myocardial scintigraphy with thallium-201 and gallium-67 in cardiac sarcoidosis. Chest. 1995;107:330–4.
4. Ohira H, Tsujino I, Yoshinaga K. (1)(8)F-Fluoro-2-deoxyglucose positron emission tomography in cardiac sarcoidosis. Eur J Nucl Med Mol Imaging. 2011;38:1773–83. doi:10.1007/s00259-011-1832-y.
5. Yamagishi H, et al. Identification of cardiac sarcoidosis with (13)N-NH(3)/(18)F-FDG PET. J Nucl Med Off Publ Soc Nucl Med. 2003;44:1030–6.
6. Tawarahara K, Kurata C, Okayama K, Kobayashi A, Yamazaki N. Thallium-201 and gallium 67 single photon emission computed tomographic imaging in cardiac sarcoidosis. Am Heart J. 1992;124:1383–4.
7. Cheng VY, et al. Impact of carbohydrate restriction with and without fatty acid loading on myocardial 18F-FDG uptake during PET: a randomized controlled trial. J Nucl Cardiol Off Publ Am Soc Nucl Cardiol. 2010;17:286–91. doi:10.1007/s12350-009-9179-5.
8. Demeure F, et al. A randomized trial on the optimization of 18F-FDG myocardial uptake suppression: implications for vulnerable coronary plaque imaging. J Nucl Med. 2014;55:1629–35. doi:10.2967/jnumed.114.138594.
9. Blankstein R, et al. Cardiac positron emission tomography enhances prognostic assessments of patients with suspected cardiac sarcoidosis. J Am Coll Cardiol. 2013. doi:10.1016/j.jacc.2013.09.022.
10. Waller AH, Blankstein R. Quantifying myocardial inflammation using F18-fluorodeoxyglucose positron emission tomography in cardiac sarcoidosis. J Nucl Cardiol Off Publ Am Soc Nucl Cardiol. 2014;21:940–3. doi:10.1007/s12350-014-9921-5.
11. Gotthardt M, Bleeker-Rovers CP, Boerman OC, Oyen WJ. Imaging of inflammation by PET, conventional scintigraphy, and other imaging techniques. J Nucl Med Off Publ Soc Nucl Med. 2010;51:1937–49. doi:10.2967/jnumed.110.076232.
12. Kaminaga T, Takeshita T, Yamauchi T, Kawamura H, Yasuda M. The role of iodine-123-labeled 15-(p-iodophenyl)-3R, S-methylpentadecanoic acid scintigraphy in the detection of local myocardial involvement of sarcoidosis. Int J Cardiol. 2004;94:99–103. doi:10.1016/j.ijcard.2003.05.012.
13. Shaw LJ, et al. Cardiovascular disease risk stratification with stress single-photon emission computed tomography technetium-99m tetrofosmin imaging in patients with the metabolic syndrome and diabetes mellitus. Am J Cardiol. 2006;97:1538–44. doi:10.1016/j.amjcard.2005.12.041.
14. Lebtahi R, et al. Somatostatin receptor scintigraphy and gallium scintigraphy in patients with sarcoidosis. J Nucl Med Off Publ Soc Nucl Med. 2001;42:21–6.
15. Morooka M, et al. Long fasting is effective in inhibiting physiological myocardial 18F-FDG uptake and for evaluating active lesions of cardiac sarcoidosis. EJNMMI Res. 2014;4:1.

Chapter 7
Multimodality Imaging of Cardiac Sarcoidosis

Ron Blankstein and Edward J. Miller

Abstract In addition to aiding the diagnosis, the role of imaging for patients with known or suspected cardiac sarcoidosis includes estimating the risk of future adverse events (prognosis) as well as identifying individuals who are more likely to benefit from immunosuppressive therapies. When considering these goals, cardiac MRI and PET both visualize different attributes of cardiac sarcoidosis and often have a complementary role. While the absence of late gadolinium enhancement on cardiac MRI has a high negative predictive value for excluding cardiac involvement and identifying patients with an excellent prognosis, PET is better suited for detecting and quantifying the amount of active myocardial inflammation. Data comparing these techniques is limited; however, we recommend that unless contraindications exist, cardiac MRI should be the preferred imaging test for screening patients who have abnormalities that are concerning for cardiac sarcoidosis. However, once disease is identified, PET should be used to determine the response to therapy as well as the burden of active extra-cardiac disease. Notably, cardiac MRI and PET are more sensitive than echocardiography and clinical criteria, and there is often no reliable reference standard to establish the diagnosis of cardiac sarcoidosis. In cases where the diagnosis cannot be clearly established (i.e. clinical and imaging findings which support cardiac sarcoidosis despite the absence of a biopsy), these imaging tests remain useful for informing prognosis as well as guiding therapies.

R. Blankstein, MD, FACC (✉)
Non-invasive Cardiovascular Imaging Program, Department of Medicine
(Cardiovascular Division) and Department of Radiology, Brigham
and Women's Hospital, Harvard Medical School, Shapiro Room
5096 75 Francis Street, Boston, MA 02115, USA
e-mail: rblankstein@partners.org

E.J. Miller, MD, PhD
Section of Cardiovascular Medicine, Boston University School of Medicine,
88 E. Newton Street, Boston, MA 02118, USA

© Springer International Publishing Switzerland 2015
A.M. Freeman, H.D. Weinberger (eds.), *Cardiac Sarcoidosis:*
Key Concepts in Pathogenesis, Disease Management, and Interesting Cases,
DOI 10.1007/978-3-319-14624-9_7

Introduction

The evaluation and management of patients with cardiac sarcoidosis requires an understanding of the role, strengths, and limitations of various different imaging modalities. Importantly, no single imaging technique can be used to reliably assess all patients with suspected or known cardiac involvement. Instead, clinicians and imagers often need to select the best available testing option to answer a particular question for a given patient. Ultimately, optimal patient management requires a careful integration of data from various different sources as well as an understanding of the implications of various imaging findings, particularly with respect to diagnosis and prognosis.

When considering what test to choose, it is important to define the role of non-invasive imaging in evaluating and managing patients with cardiac sarcoidosis (Fig. 7.1):

1. Diagnosis – Establish the presence or absence of cardiac involvement.
2. Prognosis – Identify patients who have a high (or low) risk of adverse events.
3. Identify patients who are most likely to benefit from immunosuppressive therapies.
4. Follow response to therapy.

With respect to the above goals, there is often a complementary value when combining data from various imaging modalities. For instance, information from both cardiac PET and MRI can be used to more confidently assess the likelihood of cardiac involvement. Each of these tests can image different aspects of cardiac disease making the combined findings from these two techniques particularly valuable.

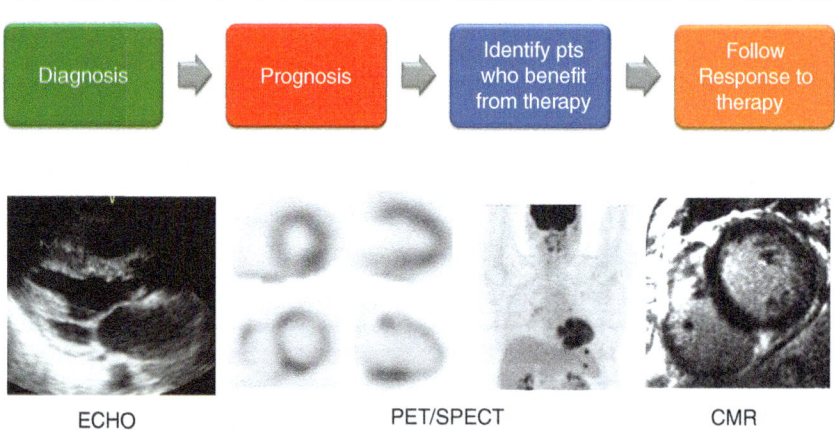

Fig. 7.1 The role of imaging in cardiac sarcoidosis

Such a hybrid approach may be especially important when the findings of any one of these tests provides inconclusive results, or when the diagnosis is challenging to establish (e.g. isolated cardiac involvement).

This chapter will discuss the role and importance of cardiac imaging in evaluating patients with known or suspected cardiac sarcoidosis. The chapter will discuss how to select among the various existing testing options as well as how to use the results provided by these tests in patient management.

When Is Advanced Multimodality Imaging Needed in a Patient with Suspected Cardiac Sarcoidosis?

The incidence of systemic sarcoidosis is increasing, and the death rate from sarcoidosis has increased 51 % from 1988 to 2007 [1]. The majority of these potentially preventable deaths in patients with sarcoidosis are from cardiac causes, but a significant percentage of patients who die of cardiac sarcoidosis have no pre-mortem symptoms [2]. Therefore, it is important to screen for cardiac involvement in patients with sarcoidosis in hopes to identify and treat patients at highest risk of adverse cardiac events. This section will explore which patients should be evaluated by advanced multimodality imaging for cardiac sarcoidosis.

A number of studies have attempted to identify the percentage of patients with sarcoidosis who have cardiac involvement. These studies are confounded by the lack of a gold standard for the diagnostic criteria for cardiac sarcoidosis. For example, the 1993 and 2006 versions of the Japanese Ministry of Health and Welfare Diagnostic Criteria for cardiac sarcoidosis are insensitive for detecting cardiac involvement and do not risk stratify patients in the same manner as advanced imaging with either cardiac MRI (CMR) [3] or ^{18}F-flurodeoxyglucose PET [4, 5]. In addition, unless a positive endomyocardial biopsy is obtained, these criteria require the presence of extra cardiac disease in order to establish the diagnosis of cardiac sarcoidosis. Therefore, it is extremely difficult to establish the diagnosis of isolated cardiac sarcoidosis using these criteria.

While there is no prospective data identifying the optimal screening strategy among patients with sarcoidosis, there is data to suggest that non-invasive screening strategies including evaluations of symptoms (palpitations, syncope, or pre-syncope), ECG (AV block, right bundle branch block, left anterior fascicular block, left posterior fascicular block, abnormal T waves), echocardiography (LVEF < 45 %, regional wall motion abnormalities, left ventricular hypertrophy, focal aneurysms), or Holter monitor (PVCs > 10/h, non-sustained ventricular tachycardia, Supraventricular tachycardia) can be used as a trigger to pursue advanced imaging with CMR and/or FDG PET with myocardial perfusion imaging.

The most common indication for screening patients with extra-cardiac sarcoidosis is the development of new cardiac signs or symptoms. Three studies have evaluated the utility of abnormal results on screening strategies to predict CMR and FDG PET abnormalities in patients with extra-cardiac sarcoidosis.

Mehta et al. [6] evaluated the ability of symptoms, ECG, echocardiogram, and Holter monitoring to predict the presence of abnormal imaging findings by either CMR or FDG PET. In their cohort of 62 patients with biopsy-proven extra-cardiac sarcoidosis, cardiac symptoms (46 vs. 5 %), abnormal Holter monitoring (50 vs. 3 %), and abnormal echocardiogram findings (25 vs. 5 %) were more common in patients who had abnormal CMR or FDG PET studies. Nearly half (47 %) of patients had some abnormality on baseline screening testing, and of those with abnormal screening testing 88 % had abnormal FDG PET and 36 % had abnormal CMR studies. Collectively, the sensitivity of any of the above screening variables to detect cardiac sarcoidosis was 100 % and the specificity was 87 %. Freeman et al. [7] used a more detailed screening regimen incorporating ECG (resting and signal averaged), echocardiogram, electrophysiology study (if performed), and nuclear stress testing to retrospectively evaluate 70 patients with systemic sarcoidosis. They found increasing numbers of abnormal screening studies were associated with a greater likelihood of abnormal CMR or FDG PET results, and that the absence of abnormal screening results lead to a lower rate (2/18, 11 %) of abnormal advanced imaging. In both the studies by Mehta and Freeman, a greater number of abnormal screening tests lead to an increased likelihood of abnormal advanced imaging. Consistent with these findings, recent data from a small study has showed that among patient without cardiac symptoms and normal LV systolic function on echocardiography, the rate of abnormal findings on CMR imaging was low (13 %) [8]. Collectively, the above data can be used to support the use of cardiac symptoms, abnormal ECGs, or abnormal echocardiographic findings for pursuing advanced imaging testing in patients with extra-cardiac sarcoidosis. The Heart Rhythm Society Expert Consensus Statement on Arrhythmias Associated with Cardiac sarcoidosis has also endorsed this strategy [9].

There are certain other clinical scenarios that should prompt an evaluation for cardiac sarcoidosis even when there is no prior history of sarcoidosis. These include new onset unexplained advanced heart block in adults under 60 years of age and/or unexplained ventricular tachycardia. Among patients with new unexplained heart block, cardiac sarcoidosis may be present in 25–34 % [10, 11]. Furthermore, numerous reports have described unexplained sustained monomorphic ventricular tachycardia (VT) as the initial presenting symptom of cardiac sarcoidosis. In these scenarios, if the patient does not have known extra-cardiac sarcoidosis then the use of chest CT or whole-body FDG PET/CT imaging may identify previously clinically silent extra-cardiac sarcoidosis (i.e. hilar/mediastinal lymphadenopathy) that is more amenable to biopsy than the heart. While the identification of extra-cardiac sarcoidosis significantly increases the likelihood of cardiac sarcoidosis, it is important to recognize that isolated cardiac sarcoidosis – whereby the disease is confined only to the heart – is likely significantly under diagnosed and may carry a worse prognosis. Therefore, the absence of extra-cardiac disease cannot be used to exclude the possibility of cardiac sarcoidosis.

In summary, our recommendations for screening for cardiac sarcoidosis include:

1. All patients with sarcoidosis should undergo a regular clinical evaluation which includes prompting for any new cardiac signs or symptoms. In addition, all patients should be screened with ECGs as part of their clinical care. Among selected patients, Holter monitoring can be performed if symptoms warrant. In addition, among selected patients, echocardiography can also be performed, realizing it is insensitive for detecting cardiac involvement or for predicting abnormal CMR or FDG PET findings (see next section).
2. Any abnormal screening test, new cardiac sign or symptom, or high clinical suspicion, particularly unexplained heart block or VT, should prompt further evaluation with CMR and/or FDG PET with myocardial perfusion imaging.

However, it is important to acknowledge that the role of wider screening of all patients with sarcoidosis with CMR (which, as discussed below, is likely a better screening test than PET given its higher sensitivity and lower cost) remains unknown. On one hand, such an approach will identify more patients who have cardiac involvement. On the other hand, it is unknown if identifying and treating clinically silent disease will lead to any improvement in patient outcomes, and whether such approaches will be cost effective, particularly when also considering the cost of downstream testing that may occur.

Role of Multimodality Imaging in the Diagnosis of Cardiac Sarcoidosis

Imaging plays a critical role in the diagnosis of cardiac sarcoidosis and is particularly important due to the insensitivity of cardiac biopsy and the imprecision of clinical criteria in diagnosing cardiac sarcoidosis. A number of imaging techniques have been used to evaluate for cardiac sarcoidosis, including echocardiography, nuclear perfusion imaging, imaging of inflammation (FDG PET and gallium-67), and cardiac MRI (CMR). While most of these techniques have been reviewed in other chapters in this book, this section will provide a multi-modality overview of how these tests are used to diagnose cardiac sarcoidosis. In addition, we will present an algorithm for the use of advanced multimodality imaging for the evaluation of cardiac sarcoidosis, highlighting the complementary aspects of CMR and FDG PET with myocardial perfusion imaging (MPI).

Echocardiography

Echocardiography has been used to evaluate patients for sarcoidosis since the mid-1980s. Classic echocardiographic patterns for sarcoidosis involving the heart include the presence of basal septal thinning, depressed left ventricular ejection fraction, regional wall motion abnormalities (RWMAs), focal hypertrophy, or left ventricular aneurysms. These findings are neither sensitive nor specific for cardiac sarcoidosis and do not correlate well with CMR or FDG PET with MPI. For example, Mehta et al. found echocardiographic abnormalities in only 25 % of the patients who exhibited CMR or FDG PET evidence of cardiac sarcoidosis [6] and Freeman et al. determined a negative predictive value of only 32 % for echocardiography [7]. This corresponds to unpublished data from our own group suggesting that in patients with suspected cardiac sarcoidosis, echocardiograms are normal in as many as a quarter of patients who have FDG PET studies with abnormal perfusion and half of patients who have abnormal FDG uptake (Miller et al. unpublished data). Thus in our opinion, the low sensitivity and negative predictive value of echocardiography when compared to other techniques make it less suitable for use as a screening test for cardiac sarcoidosis, particularly among patients who have any of the aforementioned abnormalities that warrant screening.

Nuclear Imaging Techniques

Historically, nuclear imaging techniques such as thallium-201 or gallium-67 scintigraphy have been used to evaluate for abnormal cardiac perfusion/scar or inflammation, respectively. However, these have been supplanted by newer techniques. Specifically, PET perfusion tracers (rubidium-82 and N-13 ammonia) have increased sensitivity and specificity compared to thallium-201 or technetium-99m for detection of perfusion defects. Among patients with cardiac sarcoidosis, such defect may be due to scar and/or marked inflammation resulting in compression of the microvasculature. For the detection of cardiac inflammation, ^{18}F-flurodeoxyglucose has superior diagnostic performance compared to gallium-67. Therefore, FDG PET performed with MPI has become the standard of care for nuclear imaging evaluation of cardiac sarcoidosis since it can evaluate both pathological processes of cardiac sarcoidosis (scar and inflammation).

Appropriate pre-scan patient preparation is essential in order to suppress the uptake of FDG from normal myocardium. Further details regarding this are available in Chap. 6. Based on the experience of our centers we suggest one of the following protocols:

- A high fat/low carbohydrate diet for two meals prior to the scan followed by a fast of at least 4 h
- A high fat/low carbohydrate diet followed by a fast of at least 12 h

Prior to imaging, it should be confirmed that the patients were able correctly follow the diet/preparation instruction.

The acquisition protocol for FDG PET with MPI for cardiac sarcoidosis is discussed in detail in Chap. 6 and is shown in Fig. 7.2. The study begins with a resting myocardial perfusion imaging study. When available, PET resting MPI (Rb-82 or N-13 NH$_3$) is preferable, but SPECT MPI (Tc-99m) can also be performed, and should be combined with attenuation correction when available. Subsequently, the patient is injected with 10–12 mCi of F18- FDG. Following an uptake period of 90 min 3-D FDG PET acquisition of the heart and whole body is performed.

7 Multimodality Imaging of Cardiac Sarcoidosis

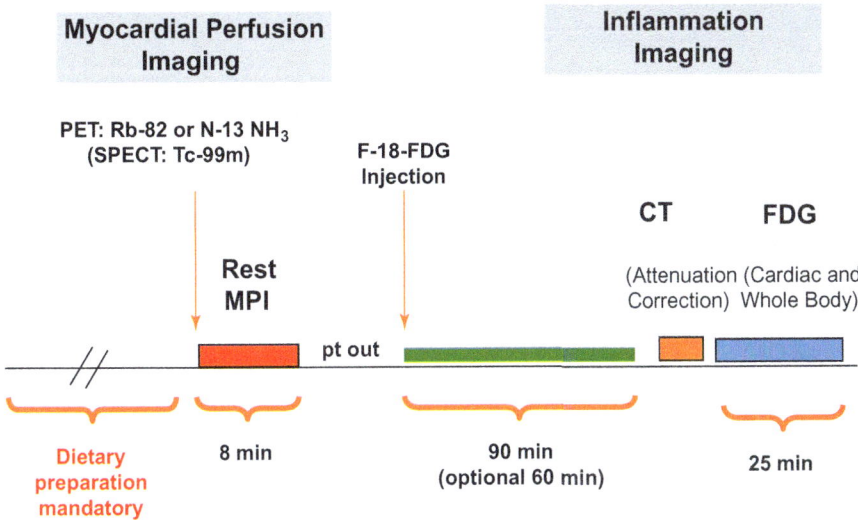

Fig. 7.2 Example of a FDG PET plus MPI protocol for cardiac sarcoidosis. Further details are provided in the text as well as in Chap. 7

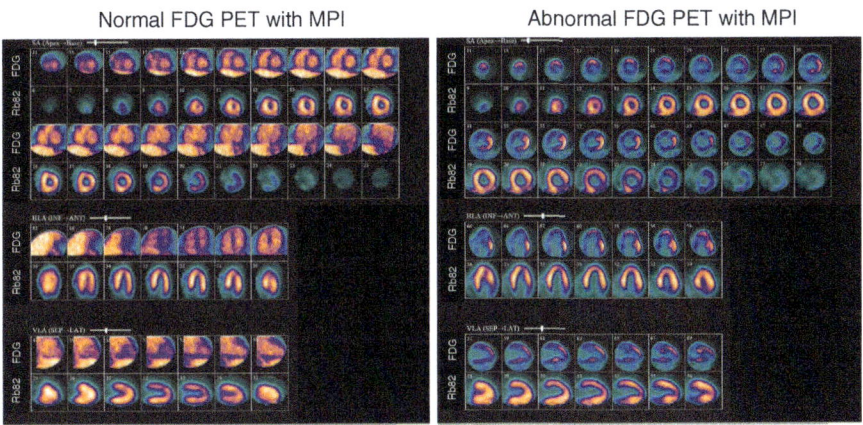

Fig. 7.3 Example of FDG PET with MPI images for the evaluation of cardiac sarcoidosis. (*Left*) Normal pattern for fasting FDG images in the heart, showing no myocardial uptake, but faint FDG signal present in the LV blood pool. Rb82 perfusion is normal. (*Right*) Abnormal FDG PET with MPI showing a focal area of FDG uptake with greater intensity than LV blood pool in the basal lateral/infero-lateral walls. In addition, there is a focal basal infero-lateral perfusion defect on the Rb82 images. This highlights the complementary information gained by use of FDG (inflammation) and Rb82 (scar) imaging for the evaluation of cardiac sarcoidosis

The interpretation of FDG PET with MPI studies includes an evaluation of both perfusion and FDG uptake (Fig. 7.3). Perfusion defects are described using a traditional 0–4 grading scale for severity and 17-segment model for location. Abnormal FDG uptake is described as a focal or focal-on-diffuse area of the myocardial uptake

Rest Perfusion	FDG	Frequency	Example Perfusion	Example FDG	Interpretation / Comment
Normal perfusion and metabolism					
Normal	Normal (negative)	32 (27%)	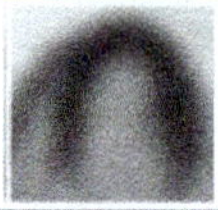		Normal
Normal	Diffuse (non-specific)	15 (12%)	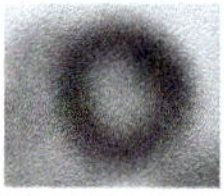	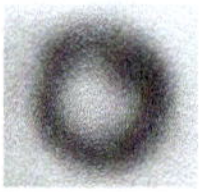	Diffuse FDG most likely due to failure to suppress FDG from normal myocardium
Abnormal perfusion or metabolism					
Normal	Focal	20 (17%)	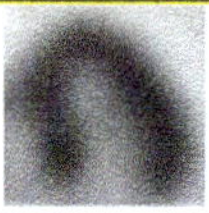	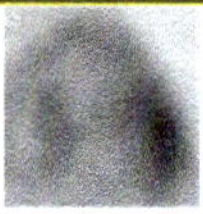	Nonspecific pattern; focal increase in FDG may represent early disease vs. normal variant
Positive	Negative	17 (14%)	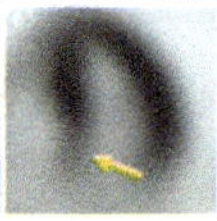		Rest perfusion defect may represent scar from cardiac sarcoidosis or other etiologies
Abnormal perfusion and metabolism					
Positive	Focal increase ("mismatch patter")	23 (19%)	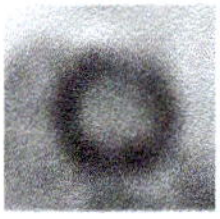	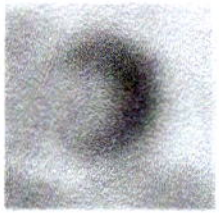	Presence of active inflammation ± scar in the same location
Positive	Focal on diffuse	6 (5%)	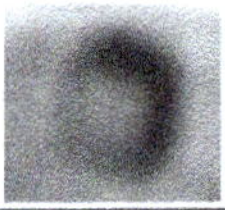	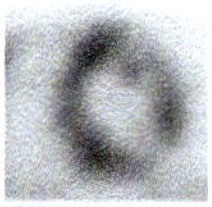	Similar to above but also areas of inability to suppress FDG from normal myocardium vs. diffuse inflammation
Positive	Focal increase (different area)	5 (4%)	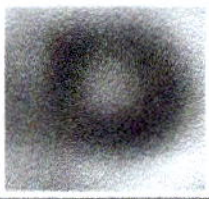	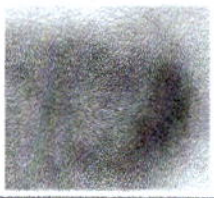	Presence of the both scar and inflammation but in different segments

Fig. 7.4 Classification of cardiac PET/CT perfusion and metabolism imaging. (With permission from Elsevier Publication. Source: Blankstein et al. [5])

with intensity greater than the left ventricular blood pool (see Fig. 7.4 for examples). In addition, it is important to describe whether there are focal areas of increased FDG uptake involving the right ventricle. Whole body FDG imaging using a large field of view from the base of the skull to the mid-thigh level should be performed in order to evaluate for extra-cardiac sarcoidosis.

While cardiac sarcoidosis may cause isolated FDG uptake without any perfusion defects, or in more advance stages of disease, resting perfusion defects without any FDG uptake, the most characteristic finding is a perfusion/metabolism "mismatch" whereby areas of increased FDG also exhibit a resting perfusion defect. It is noteworthy that such a mismatch pattern can also occur in patients with hibernating myocardium, and thus when the diagnosis of cardiac sarcoidosis is suspected based on such PET findings, it may be necessary to rule out the presence of obstructive coronary artery disease (CAD). Nevertheless, at times, there are challenging cases where CAD and cardiac sarcoidosis can both be present.

Recently, newer methods of quantitative interpretation of FDG uptake including the volume of inflammation [12] and integrated volume-intensity [4] have been described. Such measures are most useful when comparing scans in order to follow response to therapy, but may also enhance the standardization of interpretation among centers.

While there are wide ranges of estimates for the sensitivity of FDG PET with MPI for detecting cardiac sarcoidosis, these estimates are rather misleading given the lack of a reference gold standard criteria and the fact that imaging is more sensitive for detecting disease than the Japanese criteria. With these important limitations in mind, a recent meta-analysis involving a total of 164 patients from 7 studies described a sensitivity of 89 % and specificity of 78 % when compared against the 2006 JMHW criteria [13]. However, the reduced specificity of PET in these studies may be due to the fact that it is more sensitive than the reference criteria against which it was compared.

Cardiac MRI

Cardiac MRI is also an important and useful advanced cardiac imaging technique used for the evaluation for cardiac sarcoidosis. CMR is a highly accurate technique to evaluate cardiac structure and function, and it can be used to define morphological features of cardiac sarcoidosis analogous to echocardiography (e.g. regional wall motion abnormalities, wall thinning, hypertrophy, LV systolic dysfunction, and focal aneurysms). However, the major role for CMR in the diagnosis of cardiac sarcoidosis lies in the evaluation of late gadolinium enhancement (LGE) whereby T1 weighted inversion recovery images are acquired ~10 min following the administration of intravenous gadolinium. Gadolinium is an extracellular contrast agent that has a rapid washout from normal areas of myocardium. However, in patients with cardiac sarcoidosis, the presence of scar or intense inflammation can expand the extracellular space and result in slower washout of gadolinium and thus areas of increased T1 signal enhancement. Such areas of LGE – which commonly are sub-epciardial or midwall in location – may be seen even when there are no regional wall motion abnormalities and normal wall thickness. As a result, in patients with suspected cardiac sarcoidosis, the presence of LGE is more sensitive than echocardiography and perfusion imaging for the detection of scar formation.

While the typical pattern of LGE in cardiac sarcoidosis is a non-transmural pattern involving either the sub-epicardial and/or mid-myocardial walls (Fig. 7.4), patterns of subendocardial or transmural LGE (which may mimic common CAD patterns) have been described as well.

Similar to FDG PET, estimates of the accuracy of CMR to diagnose cardiac sarcoidosis are hampered by a lack of gold standard. The original report of the diagnostic accuracy of CMR for cardiac sarcoidosis showed a sensitivity of 100 % and specificity of 78 % versus the JMHW criteria [14] with the low specificity a consequence of comparison versus the insensitive JMHW criteria. This superiority of CMR for diagnosing cardiac involvement in sarcoidosis was borne out by Patel et al. who showed a greater than 2x increase in cardiac sarcoidosis diagnosis versus JMHW criteria, leading to a significant improvement in prognostication of adverse events by CMR when compared to JMHW criteria [14].

There is only a single small study that has directly compared CMR and PET, the results of which support the complementary value of these two techniques. In this study, Ohira et al. [15] evaluated 21 consecutive patients with suspected cardiac sarcoidosis who underwent both exams and found that 5 were negative by both modalities and 8 were positive by both. Interestingly, 8 patients had discordant findings: 7 had only PET abnormalities while 1 had only CMR abnormalities. Among the 8 (38 %) patients who were categorized as having CS by JMHW criteria, 3 had abnormal findings by only one modality while 5 had abnormalities on both. This study was underpowered to detect significant differences in diagnostic accuracy between these techniques, but has been incorrectly quoted by some to suggest that PET may have a higher sensitivity based on a non-significant, numerically higher sensitivity for PET [7 out of 8] than CMR [6 out of 8] (Fig. 7.5).

Selecting the Right Test

Recommendations regarding the optimal multimodality imaging strategy for the diagnosis of cardiac sarcoidosis are hampered by a lack of prospective data. Possible strategies include use of either CMR or FDG PET with MPI in isolation or a complementary approach where both techniques are applied to every patient. Any approach should take into account the strengths and limitations of each institution's imaging capabilities and experience. Our approach is outlined in Fig. 7.6. In patients with suspected cardiac sarcoidosis based on screening criteria or clinical scenario outlined in the previous section, a 'CMR first' strategy can be employed if the patient is eligible for a CMR based on lack of a cardiac device and appropriate renal function. Consistent with recent HRS Consensus Statement criteria [9], positive CMR findings in patients with diagnosed extra-cardiac sarcoidosis are satisfactory to diagnose a patient with cardiac sarcoidosis and warrant consideration of primary prevention ICD implantation. In patients who cannot obtain a CMR, those who have inconclusive CMR results, or in whom the CMR is negative but there is a high clinical suspicion for cardiac sarcoidosis, FDG PET with MPI should then be pursued in order to better clarify the likelihood of cardiac sarcoidosis.

Our recommendation of a 'CMR first' imaging strategy is based on: (1) improved sensitivity and higher negative predictive value (NPV) of CMR; (2) lack of radiation exposure; (3) lower cost. CMR may also have a small advantage in that it does not require dietary preparation. While FDG PET imaging may lead to non-diagnostic results when there is inadequate suppression of FDG from the normal myocardium, when using CMR for screening, non-specific results can also be encountered (e.g. small foci of LGE which could also be due to other etiologies such as prior myocarditis). Therefore, regardless of which imaging testing is selected initially, there is

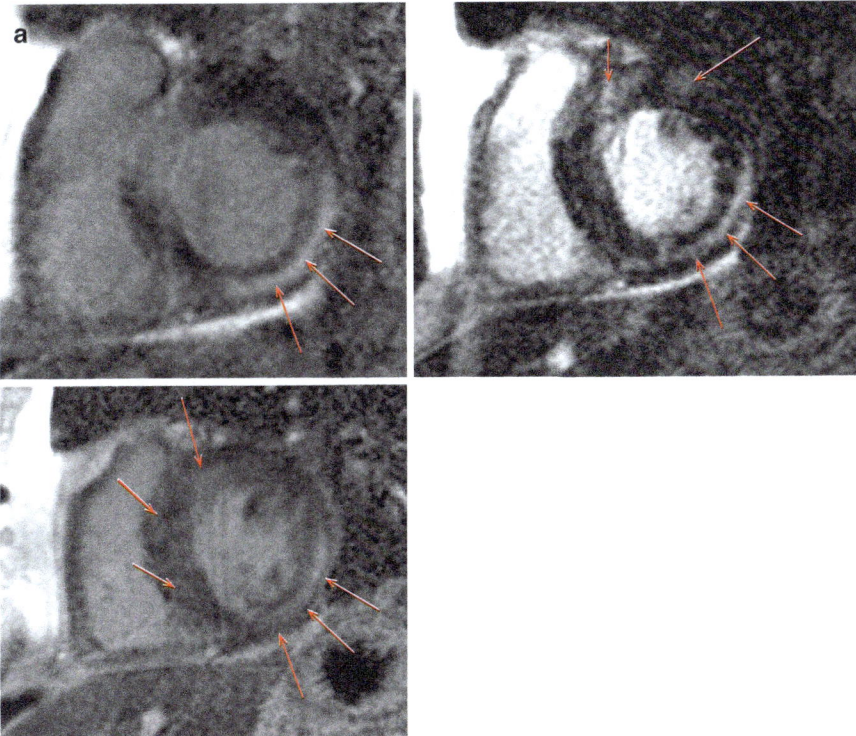

Fig. 7.5 Forty-eight year old male who presented with ventricular tachycardia following exercise. There was no history to support the diagnosis of myocarditis and cardiac enzymes were negative. (**a**) Cardiac MRI showed a large amount of mid wall and sub-epicardial late gadolinium enhancement involving the basal and mid inferolateral wall as well as the basal and mid anteroseptum, inferoseptum, and anterior wall. (*red arrows*) Endomyocardial biopsy was negative and showed no granulomatous inflammation. (**b**) PET FDG demonstrated a large amount of increased FDG uptake, which was most prominent in the basal inferior, inferolateral, and inferoseptal walls. Following 5 months of steroid therapy there was a marked reduction in the extent and intensity of FDG uptake (**c**) as well as a reduction in the burden of ventricular arrhythmias. The patient did not have any extra cardiac disease. In this case, despite a negative endomyocardial biopsy, the patient was diagnosed with isolated cardiac sarcoidosis

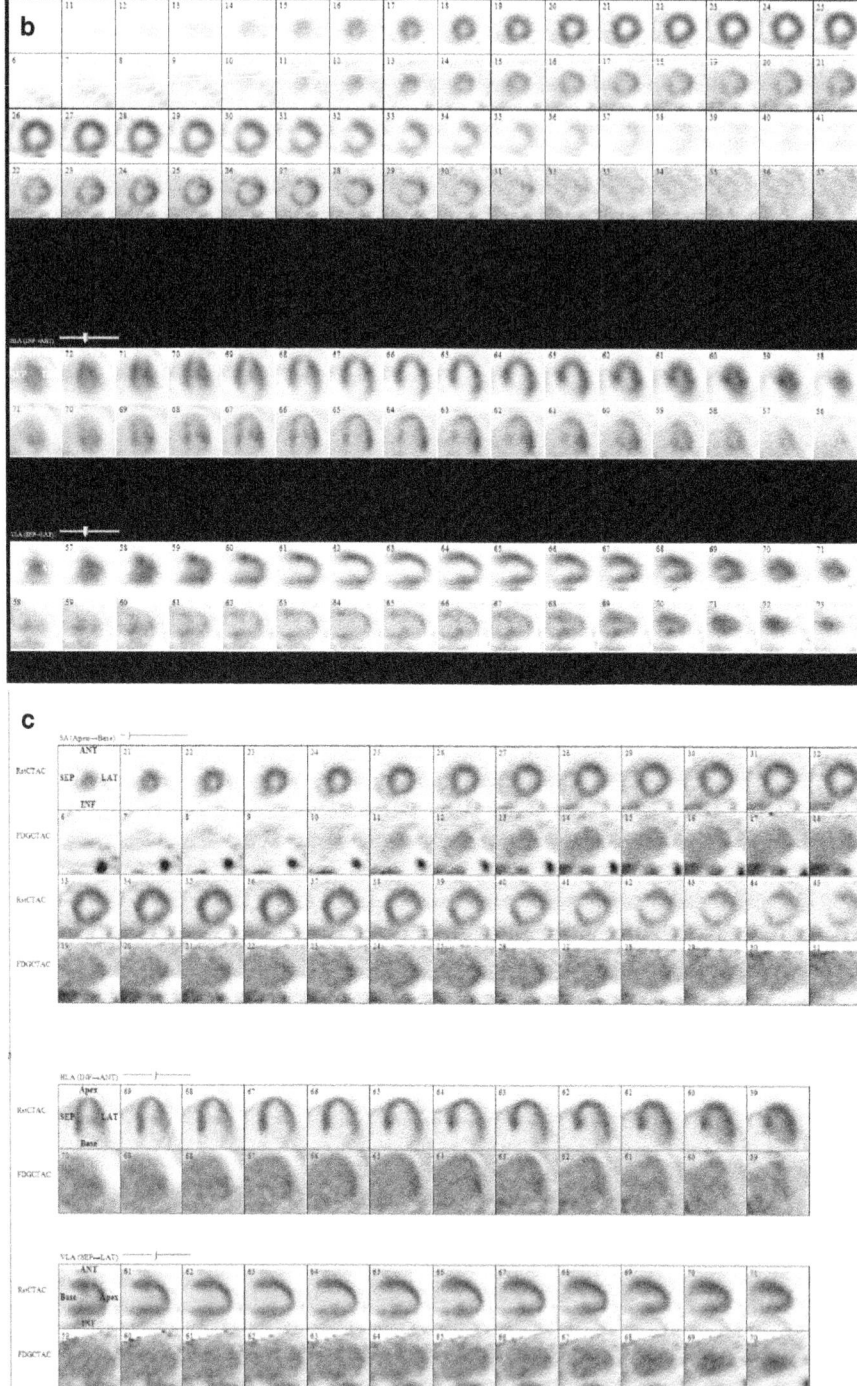

Fig. 7.5 (continued)

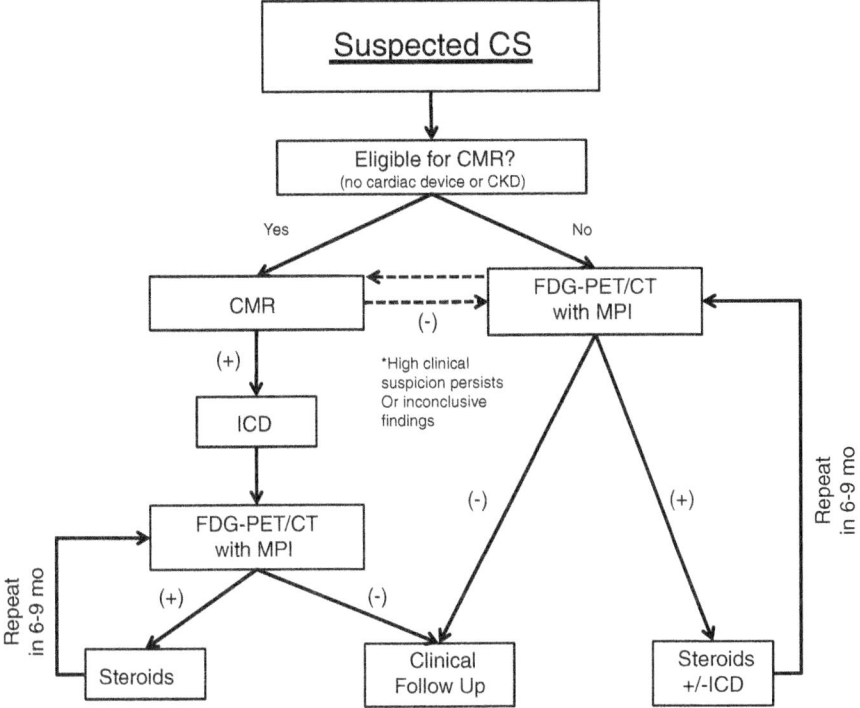

Fig. 7.6 Use of advanced multimodality imaging for the evaluation of cardiac sarcoidosis

always a possibility that due to inconclusive findings, additional complementary imaging may be helpful.

Another caveat to CMR imaging is that in early stages of disease, CMR may be negative while PET may demonstrate focal uptake of FDG. While some CMR techniques such at T2 weighted imaging or T2 mapping may enable the identification of early disease, these sequences are challenging to perform and are generally inferior to FDG imaging for detecting inflammation. Given the above considerations, when available and in the absence of contraindications, it is reasonable to employ a concomitant imaging strategy with both CMR and PET (FDG and MPI) strategy in patients with suspected cardiac sarcoidosis. However, the cost and clinical effectiveness of this approach remain to be determined.

Role of Multimodality Imaging in Establishing Prognosis of Cardiac Sarcoidosis

Emerging data has shown that both cardiac MRI and PET provide information that can be used to identify which patients with suspected cardiac sarcoidosis have the highest risk of adverse events such as cardiac death or ventricular tachycardia.

Table 7.1 Prognostic value of CMR

Study	Number/type of patients	Number of patients with LGE	Median F/U (months)	Overall number of events	Number of events in patients with no LGE	Conclusions
Patel et al. [3]	81 w/extra cardiac disease	21 (26 %)	21	8 [5 death, 2 VT, 1 AVB]	2 [1 cardiac death; 1 non-cardiac death]	(+) CMR associated with events; more sensitive than clinical criteria
Greulich et al. [20]	155 w/extra cardiac disease	39 (25 %)	31	12 [death/ SCD/ICD Rx]	1 [1 non-cardiac death]	(+) CMR is a strong predictor of potentially lethal events
Nagai et al. [8]	61 w/extra cardiac disease	8 (13 %)	50	1 [1 AVB]	2 [2 non-cardiac death]	Both patients with and w/out LGE had low event rates

Before discussing the results of these studies, it must be acknowledged that unlike the data available for other more common cardiac disease, the available data on the prognostic value of cardiac MRI and PET is limited to smaller studies. Nevertheless, this is important and useful data, particularly given the lower prevalence of cardiac sarcoidosis and the fact that for many patients with suspected cardiac sarcoidosis, the exact diagnosis may be uncertain. In such cases, it could be argued that regardless of the final diagnosis, any imaging findings that can identify high-risk patients would be clinically important and could be used to guide therapies, such as ICD's, which may offer survival advantage.

Table 7.1 summarized the results of three available studies that have examined the prognostic value of cardiac MRI. These studies, together with several other studies that are not yet published, support the fact that the presence of late enhancement on cardiac MRI is associated with a higher risk of death or ventricular tachycardia. As importantly, patients who do not have any late enhancement had an extremely low event rate, with only one cardiac event reported in three studies. Therefore, cardiac MRI may be used not only to exclude the presence of cardiac sarcoidosis in the vast majority of patients with suspected disease, but also to identify patients who have an excellent prognosis.

While most of the studies to date have categorized the CMR findings as positive or negative, one study has suggested that patients who have a greater extent of late enhancement (late gadolinium enhancement mass ≥ 20 % of LV mass) were more likely to have adverse events and were less likely to have an improvement in their left ventricular function [16].

Table 7.2 summarizes the results of two available studies to date which have examined the prognostic value of cardiac PET. Blankstein et al. found that patients who had both (a) increased myocardial inflammation (i.e. focal uptake of FDG) and (b) resting perfusion defects experienced a fourfold increase in the rate of death or ventricular

Table 7.2 Prognostic value of PET

Study	Number/types of patient	PET findings	Median F/U (months)	Overall number of events	Number of events in patients with normal perfusion/no FDG uptake	Conclusions
Blankstein et al. [5]	118 w/ known or suspected cardiac sarcoidosis	47 (40 %) normal; 34 (28 %) had abnormal perfusion AND FDG uptake	18	31 [27 VT; 8 deaths]	6 [4 VT; 2 deaths] All had LV or RV dysfunction	Increased FDG and resting perfusion defects associated with increased risk of death/VT
Ahmadian et al. [4]	31 w/known or suspected cardiac sarcoidosis	2 (6 %) normal; 12 (39 %) abnormal perfusion AND FDG uptake; Quantitative FDG volume: intensity correlated with abnormal visual FDG	450 ± 271 days	12 (3 VT; 0 deaths)	1 (CHF)	Quantitation of FDG uptake predicts events

tachycardia [5]. Importantly, the association between abnormal PET findings and adverse events persisted even after adjusting for left ventricular ejection fraction, clinical criteria, and the presence of active extra-cardiac disease [5]. In addition, the presence of focal uptake of FDG by the right ventricle was found to be associated with an extremely high event rate. Further studies are required in order to identify whether patients with RV FDG uptake represent those who have more extensive disease or if the higher rate of events in these patients is due to the involvement of more arrhythmogenic substrate.

Similar to the results of the study by Blankstein et al. recent work by Ahmadian et al. [4] also highlight the importance of FDG PET with MPI findings in determining the prognosis of patients with suspected cardiac sarcoidosis. In this study, among 31 patients with suspected sarcoidosis, 24 met clinical diagnostic criteria (including FDG PET and CMR findings) for the diagnosis of cardiac sarcoidosis. During follow up, 12 cardiac events occurred among 9 patients, and the majority of events occurred in individuals with abnormal FDG uptake.

Based on the published studies performed to date, the event rate in patients referred for cardiac PET is higher than those referred for cardiac MRI. This difference can be explained by the fact that patients referred for PET are more likely to already have an ICD (which is a contraindication for cardiac MRI) and prior history of ventricular tachycardia. In fact, the event rate observed in patients referred for cardiac PET (which is usually performed in tertiary referral centers) is similar to the event rate experienced by patients with cardiac sarcoidosis who have been treated with ICD implantation for primary or secondary prevention of sudden cardiac death [17, 18].

While there are no published studies in this regards, it seems plausible that the findings provided by cardiac MRI (which provides an estimate of the extent of scar) as well as those provided by PET imaging with FDG (which provide an estimate of the overall magnitude and extent of myocardial inflammation) may be complementary, both for diagnosing and treating disease, as well as for providing an estimate of the risk of future adverse events.

The Role of Imaging in Patients with Known Cardiac Sarcoidosis

In patients who have known cardiac sarcoidosis, there are multiple important imaging questions. First, what is the risk of developing worsening heart failure or ventricular arrhythmias/sudden cardiac death. In patients who have significant inflammation, as detected by FDG PET, a more compelling argument could be made for treatment with systemic anti-inflammatory therapies. Interestingly, Osborne et al. suggested that when such therapies result in a significant reduction in the volume or extent of myocardial inflammation, the left ventricular systolic function may improve [12]. Similarly, patients who have a higher risk of sudden cardiac death should have an even stronger consideration for ICD placement.

In addition to the above questions, other pertinent imaging questions may include assessing the left ventricular dimensions and systolic function or evaluating for aneurysms. Patients with pulmonary disease should also have an evaluation of the right heart chambers, and in selected patients the pulmonary artery systolic pressure should be estimated to evaluate for possible pulmonary hypertension. Finally, less frequently, cardiac sarcoidosis can also involve other cardiac structures such as the pericardium, the valves, or even the coronary arteries. Therefore, regardless of what imaging tests are being used, it is important to be as comprehensive as possible when imaging patients with cardiac sarcoidosis, and to recognize that no single test will be able to always provide all the clinically relevant data for this condition.

Use of Multimodality Imaging to Assess Response to Therapy

Among patients who are treated or who are being considered for treatment with systemic anti-inflammatory therapies, imaging may provide a useful mechanism to directly follow – and quantify – the response to therapy. Such an approach may allow clinicians to individualize therapies for each patient and hopefully minimize the duration of toxic therapies for some patients while signifying the need to select alternative agents in those who do not respond. Importantly, this is a unique role of imaging since, to date, there are no biomarkers that can accomplish this important task.

While case reports and small series have suggested changes in CMR LGE in response to steroid therapy in cardiac sarcoidosis, use of serial CMR imaging is frequently limited by the requirement for cardiac devices in patients with cardiac sarcoidosis. Moreover, there is no data regarding whether there are reliable and reproducible quantitative CMR techniques that can be used to assess response to therapy. Similarly, more data is needed regarding whether strain measurements on echocardiography can be used to follow response to therapy.

FDG PET with MPI can readily be used for serial examinations to guide immunosuppression therapy. However, comparison of repeated FDG PET imaging requires attention to interpretive methods. Traditionally, cardiac FDG images are displayed using a standard nuclear cardiology format that normalizes the image to the maximum intensity pixel of the study. Such an approach may be problematic for visualizing changes in the intensity and extent of FDG uptake between studies because it does not allow for precise analysis of changes in peak intensity. This can be overcome by measuring the absolute intensity of FDG uptake using multi-modality PET/CT workstations (e.g. GE AW suite; MIM vista).

The intensity of FDG uptake in PET images can be quantified using Standard Uptake Values (SUV), which are calculated as:

$$SUV = \frac{\text{Measured Activity}(kBq/ml)}{\text{Decay corrected FDG dose}(kBq) * \text{Patent weight}(g)}$$

Recent data suggest that quantification of SUVs using various methods increases the certainty of interpretation and is useful for following response to therapy. Osborne et al. evaluated the change in FDG uptake using SUV-thresholded volume measurements from repeated FDG PET imaging from 23 patients [12]. Similarly, Ahmadian et al. [4] described the utility of quantified FDG volume-intensity to demonstrate a decrease with steroid treatment. Both groups found traditional visual interpretation and measurement of maximal SUV intensity (SUVmax) did not correlate with clinical improvement or events [19] (Fig. 7.7).

While the precise role and method for quantification of SUV changes is still evolving, Table 7.3 describes the various methods of SUV quantification that have been described for use in FDG PET for cardiac sarcoidosis.

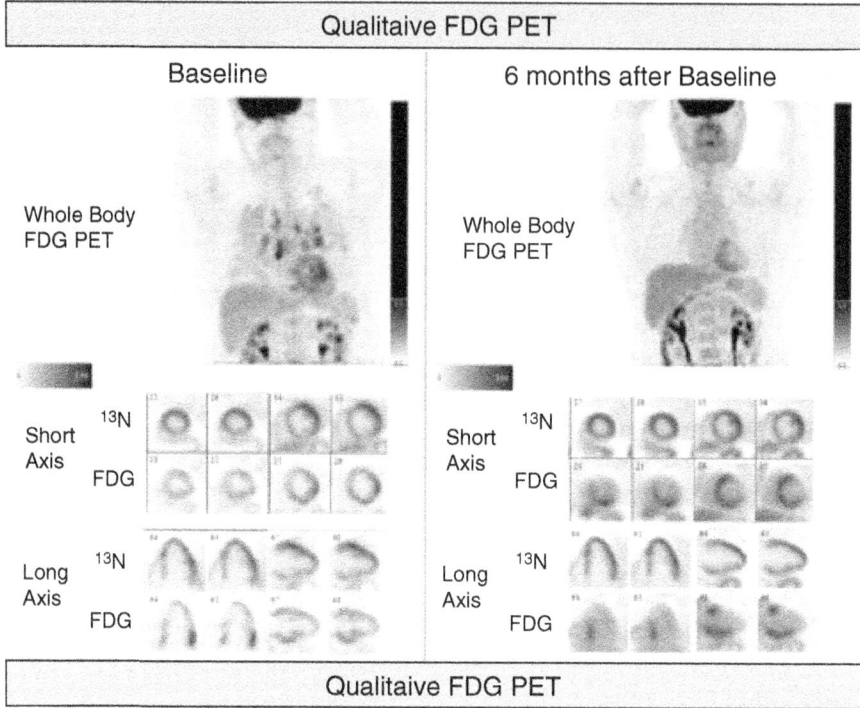

Fig. 7.7 Example of using quantitative approaches to assess changes in FDG uptake in response to therapy (Source: Waller et al. [19])

Future Directions and Important Unanswered Questions

Multimodality imaging for cardiac sarcoidosis has advanced rapidly in the past decade, due to greater access to PET scanners as well as refinement of FDG PET and cardiac MRI techniques. This has lead to the publication of important data describing the use of multimodality imaging for the diagnosis and risk stratification of patients with suspected cardiac sarcoidosis. Despite increasing levels of evidence supporting its use, further work is still needed to define the most appropriate technical application and clinical use of both CMR and FDG PET with MPI in cardiac sarcoidosis.

7 Multimodality Imaging of Cardiac Sarcoidosis

Table 7.3 Methods for quantifying FDG PET imaging for cardiac sarcoidosis

Method	Description	Study	Outcome
SUVmax	Peak measured activity	Numerous	None
Total SUV	Sum of SUVs from each cardiac segment	Okumura et al. [22]	Associated with VT
		Mc Ardle et al. [23]	
Heart: blood pool ratio	Cardiac SUVmax/aorta SUVmax	Langah et al. [24]	None
Coefficient of variance	STDEV of SUVmax for each cardiac segment/average SUV	Tahara et al. [21]	None
Volume of abnormal FDG	Volume of FDG (+) pixels using SUV threshold	Osborne et al. [12]	Reduction of this measure in response to immunosuppression is associated with improved ejection fraction
		Ahmadian et al. [4]	
Volume-intensity of abnormal FDG	Volume of FDG (+) pixels using SUV threshold × mean FDG intensity	Ahmadian et al. [4]	Associated with combined endpoint of VT/CHF/heart block

On a technical level, there needs to be increased standardization of acquisition protocols and interpretive methods for both CMR and FDG PET imaging. For example, it is unclear what role T1 (for extra-cellular volume) and T2-weighted (for edema) CMR sequences (and their quantitative mapping approaches) play in the evaluation of cardiac sarcoidosis. Interpretation of late gadolinium enhancement severity may be aided by quantification, but this approach is in its infancy. In FDG PET imaging, there is significant institutional variability in patient preparation (diet, fasting, etc.), which can limit comparison of FDG studies between institutions and may affect diagnostic accuracy. In addition, while some centers only perform a cardiac FDG acquisition (due to reimbursement and/or pre-authorization complexities), acquiring whole body FDG images is extremely beneficial and should be done routinely. Finally, further study of the optimal method of quantitative interpretation of FDG uptake is needed to overcome the inherent limitations of visual interpretation.

To improve the level of clinical evidence for both CMR and FDG PET, comparative efficacy studies are needed. Using these comparative results, new cardiac sarcoidosis diagnostic criteria can be created using multimodality imaging that is grounded in prognostic evidence. Similarly, comparative efficacy of imaging screening strategies for cardiac sarcoidosis can help define whether CMR, FDG PET with MPI, or both types of imaging should be employed in patients with suspected cardiac involvement. Lastly, further study is needed to define the best immunosuppressive treatment strategy, outlining if treatment is needed in all patients and, if so, for how long and with what agent?

In summary, both CMR and FDG PET with MPI imaging are often needed in order to fully understand the disease process in a given patient. The information gained from these studies can assist in the diagnosis, risk stratification, and following the response to treatment of patients with cardiac sarcoidosis.

Pearls of Wisdom
1. Advanced imaging with CMR (or alternatively PET) should be considered for screening selected patients with suspected cardiac sarcoidosis as these techniques are more sensitive than clinical criteria and echocardiography. Screening should be pursued for the following groups: (a) Known extra cardiac sarcoidosis with positive prior screening with ECG, Holter, or echocardiograpy – or new cardiac symptoms; (b) Patients with high clinical suspicion, particularly unexplained heart block or VT.
2. The role of wider screening of all patients with sarcoidosis is unknown. While such an approach will identify more patients who have cardiac involvement, it is unknown if identifying and treating clinically silent disease will lead to any improvement in patient outcomes, and whether such approaches will be cost effective.
3. Cardiac MRI and FDG PET both visualize different pathological attributes of cardiac sarcoidosis and likely have a complementary role for diagnosis and prognosis. Thus, when either test provides an inconclusive results the other test should be considered.
4. The absence of late gadolinium enhancement (LGE) on cardiac MRI is associated with an extremely low rate of future adverse events such as ventricular tachycardia or cardiac death. Thus, the absence of LGE can reliably exclude the presence of cardiac involvement in the vast majority of patients while identifying patients with a favorable prognosis.
5. It is recommended to assess response to anti-inflammatory therapy with serial PET FDG imaging, as some patients will experience significant (at times complete) reduction in inflammation and can be tapered off therapy while others may have no response in which case consideration of alternative treatment options is warranted.
6. When comparing serial FDG PET studies to assess the response to therapy, it is useful to quantify the amount and severity of myocardial inflammation.
7. The presence of focal uptake of FDG by the normal myocardium together with resting myocardial perfusion defects (i.e. perfusion/metabolism mismatch) identifies patients who have a higher risk of ventricular tachycardia/sudden cardiac death.
8. In some patients with perfusion / metabolism mismatch (i.e. reduced perfusion/increased FDG uptake), excluding the presence of hibernating myocardium may be needed prior to establishing the diagnosis of cardiac sarcoidosis.
9. Due to the possibility of isolated cardiac sarcoidosis, the absence of FDG uptake outside the heart cannot be used to exclude the possibility of active cardiac disease and does not decrease the future risk of ventricular tachycardia/death.

References

1. Swigris JJ, Olson AL, Huie TJ, Fernandez-Perez ER, Solomon J, Sprunger D, et al. Sarcoidosis-related mortality in the United States from 1988 to 2007. Am J Respir Crit Care Med. 2011; 183:1524–30.
2. Silverman KJ, Hutchins GM, Bulkley BH. Cardiac sarcoid: a clinicopathologic study of 84 unselected patients with systemic sarcoidosis. Circulation. 1978;58:1204–11.
3. Patel MR, Cawley PJ, Heitner JF, Klem I, Parker MA, Jaroudi WA, et al. Detection of myocardial damage in patients with sarcoidosis. Circulation. 2009;120:1969–77.
4. Ahmadian A, Brogan A, Berman J, Sverdlov AL, Mercier G, Mazzini M, et al. Quantitative interpretation of FDG PET/CT with myocardial perfusion imaging increases diagnostic information in the evaluation of cardiac sarcoidosis. J Nucl Cardiol Off Publ Am Soc Nucl Cardiol. 2014;21:925–39.
5. Blankstein R, Osborne M, Naya M, Waller A, Kim CK, Murthy VL, et al. Cardiac positron emission tomography enhances prognostic assessments of patients with suspected cardiac sarcoidosis. J Am Coll Cardiol. 2014;63:329–36.
6. Mehta D, Lubitz SA, Frankel Z, Wisnivesky JP, Einstein AJ, Goldman M, et al. Cardiac involvement in patients with sarcoidosis: diagnostic and prognostic value of outpatient testing. Chest. 2008;133:1426–35.
7. Freeman AM, Curran-Everett D, Weinberger HD, Fenster BE, Buckner JK, Gottschall EB, et al. Predictors of cardiac sarcoidosis using commonly available cardiac studies. Am J Cardiol. 2013;112:280–5.
8. Nagai T, Kohsaka S, Okuda S, Anzai T, Asano K, Fukuda K. Incidence and prognostic significance of myocardial late gadolinium-enhancement in sarcoidosis patients without cardiac manifestation. Chest. 2014;146:1064–72.
9. Birnie DH, Sauer WH, Bogun F, Cooper JM, Culver DA, Duvernoy CS, et al. HRS expert consensus statement on the diagnosis and management of arrhythmias associated with cardiac sarcoidosis. Heart Rhythm Off J Heart Rhythm Soc. 2014;11:1305–23.
10. Nery PB, Beanlands RS, Nair GM, Green M, Yang J, McArdle BA, et al. Atrioventricular block as the initial manifestation of cardiac sarcoidosis in middle-aged adults. J Cardiovasc Electrophysiol. 2014;25:875–81.
11. Kandolin R, Lehtonen J, Kupari M. Cardiac sarcoidosis and giant cell myocarditis as causes of atrioventricular block in young and middle-aged adults. Circ Arrhythm Electrophysiol. 2011;4:303–9.
12. Osborne MT, Hulten EA, Singh A, Waller AH, Bittencourt MS, Stewart GC, et al. Reduction in 18F-fluorodeoxyglucose uptake on serial cardiac positron emission tomography is associated with improved left ventricular ejection fraction in patients with cardiac sarcoidosis. J Nucl Cardiol. 2014;21:166–74.
13. Youssef G, Leung E, Mylonas I, Nery P, Williams K, Wisenberg G, et al. The use of 18F-FDG PET in the diagnosis of cardiac sarcoidosis: a systematic review and metaanalysis including the Ontario experience. J Nucl Med Off Publ Soc Nucl Med. 2012;53:241–8.
14. Smedema J-P, Snoep G, van Kroonenburgh MP, van Geuns R-J, Dassen WR, Gorgels AP, et al. Evaluation of the accuracy of gadolinium-enhanced cardiovascular magnetic resonance in the diagnosis of cardiac sarcoidosis. J Am Coll Cardiol. 2005;45:1683–90.
15. Ohira H, Tsujino I, Ishimaru S, Oyama N, Takei T, Tsukamoto E, et al. Myocardial imaging with 18F-fluoro-2-deoxyglucose positron emission tomography and magnetic resonance imaging in sarcoidosis. Eur J Nucl Med Mol Imaging. 2008;35:933–41.
16. Ise T, Hasegawa T, Morita Y, Yamada N, Funada A, Takahama H, et al. Extensive late gadolinium enhancement on cardiovascular magnetic resonance predicts adverse outcomes and lack of improvement in LV function after steroid therapy in cardiac sarcoidosis. Heart. 2014;100:1165–72.

17. Betensky BP, Tschabrunn CM, Zado ES, Goldberg LR, Marchlinski FE, Garcia FC, et al. Long-term follow-up of patients with cardiac sarcoidosis and implantable cardioverter-defibrillators. Heart Rhythm Off J Heart Rhythm Soc. 2012;9:884–91.
18. Schuller JL, Zipse M, Crawford T, Bogun F, Beshai J, Patel AR, et al. Implantable cardioverter defibrillator therapy in patients with cardiac sarcoidosis. J Cardiovasc Electrophysiol. 2012;23: 925–9.
19. Waller AH, Blankstein R. Quantifying myocardial inflammation using F18-fluorodeoxyglucose positron emission tomography in cardiac sarcoidosis. J N Cardiol Off Publ Am Soc Nucl Cardiol. 2014;21:940–3.
20. Greulich S, Deluigi CC, Gloekler S, Wahl A, Zürn C, Kramer U, et al. CMR imaging predicts death and other adverse events in suspected cardiac sarcoidosis. JACC Cardiovasc Imaging. 2013;6:501–11.
21. Tahara N, et al. Heterogeneous myocardial FDG uptake and the disease activity in cardiac sarcoidosis. JACC Cardiovasc Imaging. 2010;3:1219–28.
22. Okumura W, et al. Usefulness of fasting 18F-FDG PET in identification of cardiac sarcoidosis. J Nucl Med 2004;45:1989–98.
23. Mc Ardle BA, et al. Is There an Association Between Clinical Presentation and the Location and Extent of Myocardial Involvement of Cardiac Sarcoidosis as Assessed by 18F-Fluorodoexyglucose Positron Emission Tomography? Circ Cardiovasc Imaging 2013;6: 617–26.
24. Langah R, Spicer K, Gebregziabher M, Gordon L. Effectiveness of prolonged fasting 18f-FDG PET-CT in the detection of cardiac sarcoidosis. J Nucl Cardiol 2009;16:801–10.

Chapter 8
Invasive Procedures and Endomyocardial Biopsy

Darlene Kim and William H. Sauer

Abstract While epicardial coronary involvement directly from sarcoidosis is rare, vasculitis is more common, and overall inflammation may create a milieu for the development of coronary disease. More common is the need for tissue diagnosis for the confirmation of a clinical scenario which suggests myocardial involvement by sarcoidosis granulomatous infiltration. While endomyocardial biopsy is the "gold standard" for a diagnosis of myocardial sarcoidosis, it remains a challenging procedure to capture the affected tissue owing to the patchy nature of the disease. Concomitant electrophysiologic or imaging studies can augment the likelihood of gathering affected tissue, but biopsy sensitivity still remains relatively low. As such, invasive study is certainly useful, but routine use is likely less in line with current standard practice.

Cardiac Catheterization

Epicardial coronary artery involvement in sarcoidosis is rare, however, can be seen as a granulomatous vasculitis. Coronary artery sarcoidosis has been confirmed on autopsy, and a case of biopsy-proven coronary artery sarcoidosis presenting as acute coronary syndrome has been reported [1, 2]. Where there is a suspicion of atherosclerotic coronary artery disease, or regional myocardial wall motion or perfusion abnormalities, diagnostic coronary angiography may be useful.

Right heart catheterization to evaluate for possible cardiac sarcoidosis associated pulmonary hypertension is the diagnostic test of choice to define pulmonary artery pressures. When pulmonary hypertension is suspected on the basis of clinical presentation or echocardiographic and other non-invasive testing, an invasive hemo-

D. Kim, MD, FACC (✉)
Division of Cardiology, Department of Medicine, National Jewish Health,
1400 Jackson St., Denver, CO 80206, USA
e-mail: kimd@njhealth.org

W.H. Sauer
Section of Cardiac Electrophysiology, Division of Cardiology,
University of Colorado Hospital, 12401 East 17th Avenue, B136,
Aurora, CO 80045, USA

dynamic assessment is warranted. Please refer to Chap. 13 regarding sarcoidosis-associated pulmonary hypertension.

Historically, right ventriculography was also used to assess right ventricular function, although its utility has essentially fallen away with the development of improved imaging modalities to quantify right ventricular function.

Electrophysiology Study

Patients with extra-cardiac sarcoidosis and signs or symptoms concerning for cardiac involvement may benefit from invasive electrophysiologic studies to clarify an arrhythmic diagnosis. In addition, information gained from the direct recording of intracardiac electrical signals can identify areas of scar consistent with granulomatous infiltration. These areas of reduced voltage can be targeted for biopsy in cases where a histological diagnosis of cardiac sarcoidosis would direct immunosuppressive therapy (see voltage guided biopsy section below).

In patients with extra-cardiac sarcoidosis and unexplained palpitations, and/or syncope, an EP study can identify an arrhythmic cause and possibly suggest a diagnosis of cardiac involvement. Inducible monomorphic ventricular tachycardia in these patients is a major diagnostic criteria for establishing cardiac involvement in the Revised JMH criteria and is included in the HRS/ACC/WASOG diagnosis for "probable cardiac sarcoidosis [3]." Therefore, ventricular stimulation for a VT induction attempt is a potential path for diagnosis of cardiac sarcoidosis in the absence of other criteria. In addition, the ability to induce VT is a risk factor for sudden death and an indication for ICD implantation for the primary's prevention of sudden death (see Chap. 12 on The role of ICD for the management of sudden death risk) [4].

Endomyocardial Biopsy: A Limited Gold Standard

Histologic diagnosis by myocardial biopsy remains the gold standard for a diagnosis of cardiac sarcoidosis. Endomyocardial biopsies demonstrating non-caseating granuloma in the heart definitively proves the diagnosis. Unfortunately, while highly specific, endomyocardial biopsies historically are not very sensitive for cardiac sarcoidosis. As a result, cardiac sarcoidosis is often treated presumptively based on clinical diagnosis alone. When the diagnosis is suspected based on a probable clinical picture in the context of confirmed systemic sarcoidosis, and supportive radiographic and ECG evidence, treatment with immunosuppressive therapy like corticosteroids is reasonable and appropriate, even despite a negative endomyocardial biopsy [1].

High Specificity, But Low Sensitivity

Unlike some infiltrative cardiomyopathies, which have relatively uniform involvement, cardiac sarcoidosis tends to have a more localized and patchy distribution. Conventional endomyocardial biopsy samples are taken under fluoroscopic guidance

Table 8.1 Recent reported incidence of major and minor complications associated with endomyocardial biopsy

Major complications	
Total	<1.0 %
Death	None
Tamponade with pericardiocentesis	0.08–0.80 %
Hemothorax or pneumothorax	None
Permanent complete AV block with permanent pacemaker needed	<0.04 %
Urgent cardiac surgery	None
Minor Complications	
Total	<5.0 %
Small pericardial effusion	0.7–1.8 %
Conduction abnormalities not requiring permanent pacemaker	0.2–3.7 %
Arrhythmia	0.2–1.1 %
Tricuspid regurgitation	0.43 %

Holzmann et al. [26], Jang et al. [27], Paul et al. [28], Yilmaz et al. [29]

from the right ventricular septal wall; however, cardiac sarcoidosis often involves other regions of myocardium. Areas such as the basal and lateral left ventricular walls, which are often affected, are more challenging to sample and are not routinely biopsied [2]. The combination of patchy distribution and conventional biopsy techniques result in sampling error, rendering the diagnostic sensitivity of standard endomyocardial biopsy quite low, generally accepted to be about 20 % at best [3]. The high false-negative biopsy rates limit the usefulness of this "gold standard."

Establishing a definitive diagnosis of cardiac sarcoidosis can be important. Recognizing cardiac sarcoidosis in the absence of other organ involvement is challenging. Distinguishing cardiac sarcoidosis from other cardiomyopathies that can mimic cardiac sarcoidosis is also critical, as an accurate diagnosis impacts treatment. Although rare, cardiac sarcoidosis has been known to mimic right ventricular dysplasia and idiopathic giant cell myocarditis [4, 5]. Studies also suggest that biopsy-proven cardiac sarcoidosis may portend a worse prognosis among patients with clinically diagnosed cardiac sarcoidosis [6].

While the risk of serious complication with conventional endomyocardial biopsy, such as right ventricular perforation, is low (under 1 %), and recent case series reported no procedure-related deaths, risks must be weighed carefully with the benefit in management, operator experience, and access to expert cardiac pathology review all in mind [7]. See Table 8.1.

AHA/ACCF/ESC Joint Statement

The joint scientific statement released by the American Heart Association, American College of Cardiology Foundation, and the European Society of Cardiology in 2007 outlines the role of endomyocardial biopsy in the diagnosis and treatment of cardiovascular disease. The statement identifies specific clinical scenarios in which

Table 8.2 Clinical scenarios where endomyocardial biopsy for cardiac sarcoidosis can be considered

Heart failure for more than 2 weeks with dilated left ventricle and new ventricular arrhythmias, second-or third-degree heart block, or failure to respond to usual care within 1–2 weeks: scenario suggests possible cardiac sarcoidosis versus giant cell myocarditis versus idiopathic granulomatous myocarditis, where diagnosis has therapeutic implications
Suspected arrhythmogenic right ventricular cardiomyopathy (ARVC): multiple case reports of cardiac sardoiosis mimicking ARVC
Young patient with unexplained second- or third-degree heart block
Unexplained ventricular arrhythmias
Strong suspicion of cardiac sarcoidosis with cardiac symptoms and equivocal non-invasive testing
Patients with diagnosis of extracardiac sarcoidosis with suspected cardiac sarcoidosis in whom diagnosis confirmation will substantially change management

Nery et al. [25], Cooper et al. [12], Greif [30]

endomyocardial biopsy is recommended because "specific myocardial disorders that have unique prognoses and treatment are seldom diagnosed by noninvasive testing" [8, 9]. Clinical scenario three directly relates to cardiac sarcoidosis. Although the statement acknowledges that the diagnostic rate for cardiac sarcoidosis is low, they recommend endomyocardial biopsy for patients who present with unexplained heart failure of greater than 3 months' duration, with a dilated left ventricle, and new ventricular arrhythmias, second-, or third-degree heart block, or failure to respond to usual care within 1–2 weeks [10]. The recommendation emphasizes the important distinction between giant cell myocarditis and cardiac sarcoidosis because early transplant is recommended in the former, and corticosteroids and possibly implantable cardiac defibrillator in the latter. In addition, despite high rates of heart block, heart failure, and arrhythmias, survival is better in patients with cardiac sarcoidosis than with idiopathic giant cell myocarditis [11] (Table 8.2).

Image-Guided Biopsy

Imaging-guided biopsies may improve the diagnostic yield and overcome the sampling error that limits the sensitivity of conventional endomyocardial biopsy. 18FDG-PET scans and cardiac MRI with delayed gadolinium-enhancement can detect areas of active inflammation and/or damage. Using these scans to direct endomyocardial sampling towards areas of tissue that may be more likely to demonstrate histopathologic evidence of sarcoidosis has been demonstrated to be effective in isolated case reports. A case in which conventional biopsy of the right ventricular septum failed to yield a diagnosis, but a repeat MRI-guided biopsy of areas of transmural delayed enhancement demonstrated diagnostic non-caseating granulomas was published by Borchert et al. [12]. A paper by Kandolin et al. describes their experience in changing diagnostic strategy in detecting isolated

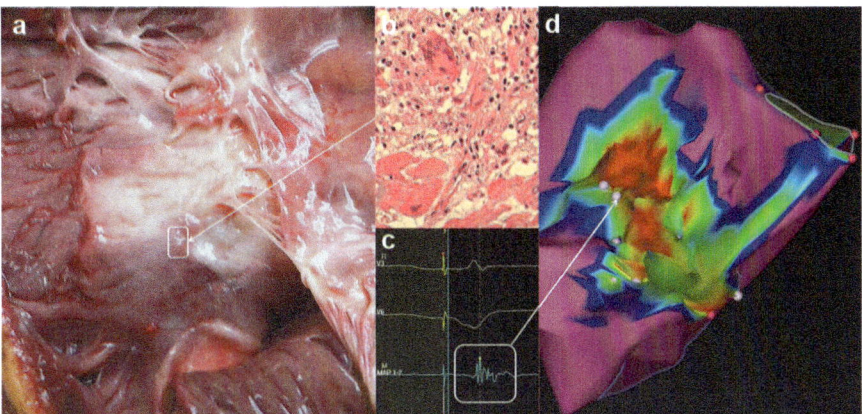

Fig. 8.1 Gross examination of an explanted heart at autopsy in a patient with cardiac sarcoidosis, revealing granulomatous myocardial scarring of the RV septum (**a**). (**b**) Shows the characteristic noncaseating granuloma infiltrating the myocardium at the border-zone with hematoxylin-eosin stained tissue at 400× power. (**c**) Shows an intracardiac electrogram recorded at a similar border-zone site. (**d**) Is the electroanatomical map of the right ventricular septum of this same patient recorded 2 years prior to autopsy. This area of reduced voltage with heterogeneous distribution of low amplitude electrograms corresponds to the myocardial scar caused by sarcoidosis related granuloma seen in the pathological examination

cardiac sarcoidosis without clinically apparent extracardiac sarcoidosis. Their experience suggests an improvement in detection rates with repeated and imaging-guided biopsies of cardiac and mediastinal lymph nodes [13].

Electroanatomical Mapping-Guided Biopsy

Three dimensional electroanatomical mapping (EAM) systems have proven to be invaluable tools as part of a strategy for mapping and ablating complex arrhythmias. In addition, these systems have also been shown to demonstrate high fidelity reconstruction of chamber dimension and quantification of viable myocardium [12]. Electrically inert tissue that results from the scar left behind after myocardial infarction or with infiltrative cardiomyopathy will be reflected by a reduced voltage recorded by a roving catheter in the endocardium or epicardial space [14]. As shown in Fig. 8.1, an area of reduced voltage recorded with EAM corresponds to myocardial scar and granulomatous infiltration as identified in histopathologic studies. The presence of mid-myocardial scar is more difficult to accurately record with a bipolar catheter; however, unipolar mapping may identify this possibility as well [15].

Electroanatomical mapping has been used in arrhythmogenic right ventricular cardiomyopathy with excellent correlation to cardiac MRI [16–19]. In addition, when endomyocardial regions of scar are identified, a bioptome can be directed to these areas for an improved diagnostic yield [22–24].

In order to perform voltage map guided biopsy, the region of scar is first identified with a roving catheter. The preferred site for biopsy is the right ventricular septum, which also represents the most common region affected by cardiac sarcoidosis. Biopsy of the epicardium and left ventricle have also been described. Again, a blind biopsy of the interventricular septum, as is common for the evaluation of other diffuse infiltrative cardiomyopathies, may not be appropriate for diagnosis of cardiac sarcoidosis given the heterogenous infiltration pattern described. Therefore, guidance with electroanatomical mapping may be more appropriate. In a study evaluating patients with right ventricular cardiomyopathy, EAM guided biopsy demonstrated a high rate of myocarditis mimicking ARVC [20]. Its use to specifically identify isolated cardiac sarcoidosis has also been demonstrated [21].

Conclusions

While the *routine* use of invasive testing cannot be supported based on current understanding, there are situations in which invasive testing provides clinically relevant information that can alter patient care that cannot be obtained with non-invasive testing. When there is a strong suspicion for cardiac sarcoidosis, especially isolated cardiac sarcoidosis, endomyocardial biopsy is appropriate and its yield may be increased by image- or electroanatomic- guided sampling.

Pearls of Wisdom

1. Cardiac catheterization for coronary angiography and right heart pressures is appropriate when there is a suspicion for coronary artery obstruction and pulmonary hypertension. Electrophysiology studies to evaluate for inducible ventricular tachycardia may be appropriate in patients who are symptomatic with palpitations and/or syncope.
2. Conventional endomyocardial biopsies have low sensitivity (less than 20 %) but high specificity, and can distinguish cardiac sarcoidosis from other pathologies, impacting treatment. Image- or electroanatomic-guided biopsies may improve diagnostic yield, but additional studies are needed.
3. Biopsy-proven cardiac sarcoidosis may identify a poorer prognosis among patients with clinical cardiac sarcoidosis (Table 8.3).

Table 8.3 Indications for EP study in patients with sarcoidosis

Rare unexplained palpitations
Risk stratification for sudden death in patients with known cardiac sarcoidosis
Unexplained syncope
Evaluation of His-Purkinje System disease

References

1. Ward E, Nazari J, Edelman R. Coronary artery vasculitis as a presentation of cardiac sarcoidosis. Circulation. 2012;125:e344–6.
2. Butany J, et al. The intricacies of cardiac sarcoidosis: a case report involving the coronary arteries and a review of the literature. Cardiovasc Pathol. 2006;15:222–7.
3. Birnie DH, Sauer WH, Bogun F, Cooper JM, Culver DA, Duvernoy CS, Judson MA, Kron J, Mehta D, Nielsen JC, Patel AR, Ohe T, Raatikainen P, Soejima K. HRS expert consensus statement on the diagnosis and management of arrhythmias associated with cardiac sarcoidosis. Heart Rhythm. 2014;11(7):1304–23.
4. Mehta D, Mori N, Goldbarg SH, Lubitz S, Wisnivesky JP, Teirstein A. Primary prevention of sudden cardiac death in silent cardiac sarcoidosis: role of programmed ventricular stimulation. Circ Arrhythm Electrophysiol. 2011;4:43–8.
5. Skhri V, Sanal S, DeLorenzo L, Arowno W, Maguire G. Cardiac sarcoidosis: a comprehensive review. Arch Med Sci. 2011;4:546–54.
6. Chang TI. Isolated cardiac sarcoidosis in heart transplantation. Transplant Proc. 2012;44(4):903–6.
7. Uemura A, Morimoto S, Hiramitsu S, Kato Y, Ito T, Hishida H. Histologic diagnostic rate of cardiac sarcoidosis: evaluation of endomyocardial iopsies. Am Heart J. 1999;138:299–302.
8. Shiraishi J, Tatsumi T, Shimoo K, Katsume A, Mani H, Kobara M, Shirayama T, Axuma A, Nakagawa M. Cardiac sarcoidosis mimicking right ventricular dysplasia. Circ J. 2003;67:169–71.
9. Sugizaki Y, Tanaka H, Imanisha J, Konishi A, Yamashita T, Shinke T, Ishida T, Kawai H, Hirata K. Isolated primary cardiac sarcoidosis presenting as acute heart failure. Intern Med. 2013;52:71–4.
10. Ardehali H, Howard D, Hariri A, Qasim A, Hare J, Baughman K, Kasper E. A positive endomyocardial biopsy result for sarcoid is associated with poor prognosis in patients with initially unexplained cardiomyopathy. Am Heart J. 2005;150:459–63.
11. From AM, Maleszewski J, Rihal C. Current status of endomyocardial biopsy. Mayo Clin Proc. 2011;86(11):1095–102.
12. Cooper LT, Baughman KL, Feldman AM, et al. The role of endomyocardial biopsy in the management of cardiovascular disease: a scientific statement from the American Heart Association, the American College of Cardiology, and the European Society of Cardiology. Circulation. 2007;116:2216–33.
13. Felker GM, Thompson RE, Hare JM, Hruban RH, Clemetson DE, Howard DL, Baughman KL, Kasper EK. Underlying causes and long-term survival in patients with initially unexplained cardiomyopathy. N Engl J Med. 2000;342:1077–84.
14. Okura Y, Dec GW, Hare JM, et al. A clinical and histopathologic comparison of cardiac sarcoidosis and idiopathic giant cell myocarditis. Am Coll Cardiol. 2003;41:322–9.
15. Borchert B, Lawrenz T, Bartelsmeir M, Rothemeyer S, Kuhn H, Stellbrink C. Utility of endomyocardial biopsy guided by delayed enhancement areas on magnetic resonance imaging in the diagnosis of cardiac sarcoidosis. Clin Res Cardiol. 2007;96:757–62.
16. Kandolin R, Lehtonen J, Graner M, Schildt J, Salmenkivi K, Kivisto S, Kupari M. Diagnosing isolated cardiac sarcoidosis. J Intern Med. 2011;270:461–8.
17. Piorkowski C, Hindricks G, Schreiber D, Tanner H, Weise W, Koch A, Gerds-Li JH, Kottkamp H. Electroanatomic reconstruction of the left atrium, pulmonary veins, and esophagus compared with the "true anatomy" on multislice computed tomography in patients undergoing catheter ablation of atrial fibrillation. Heart Rhythm. 2006;3:317–27.
18. Santangeli P, Hamilton-Craig C, Dello Russo A, Pieroni M, Casella M, Pelargonio G, Di Biase L, Smaldone C, Bartoletti S, Narducci ML, Tondo C, Bellocci F, Natale A. Imaging of scar in patients with ventricular arrhythmias of right ventricular origin: cardiac magnetic resonance versus electroanatomic mapping. J Cardiovasc Electrophysiol. 2011;22:1359–66.
19. Polin GM, Haqqani H, Tzou W, Hutchinson MD, Garcia FC, Callans DJ, Zado ES, Marchlinski FE. Endocardial unipolar voltage mapping to identify epicardial substrate in arrhythmogenic right ventricular cardiomyopathy/dysplasia. Heart Rhythm. 2011;8:76–83.

20. Corrado D, Basso C, Leoni L, Tokajuk B, Bauce B, Frigo G, Tarantini G, Napodano M, Turrini P, Ramondo A, Daliento L, Nava A, Buja G, Iliceto S, Thiene G. Three-dimensional electroanatomic voltage mapping increases accuracy of diagnosing arrhythmogenic right ventricular cardiomyopathy/dysplasia. Circulation. 2005;111:3042–50.
21. Avella A, d'Amati G, Zachara E, Musumeci F, Tondo C. Comparison between electroanatomic and pathologic findings in a patient with arrhythmogenic right ventricular cardiomyopathy/dysplasia treated with orthotopic cardiac transplant. Heart Rhythm. 2010;7:828–31.
22. Avella A, d'Amati G, Pappalardo A, Re F, Silenzi PF, Laurenzi F, DE Girolamo P, Pelargonio G, Dello Russo A, Baratta P, Messina G, Zecchi P, Zachara E, Tondo C. Diagnostic value of endomyocardial biopsy guided by electroanatomic voltage mapping in arrhythmogenic right ventricular cardiomyopathy/dysplasia. J Cardiovasc Electrophysiol. 2008;19:1127–34.
23. Avella A, d'Amati G. Diagnosis of myocarditis mimicking arrhythmogenic right ventricular cardiomyopathy: the role of endomyocardial biopsy guided by electroanatomic voltage map. J Am Coll Cardiol. 2009;54:664–5; author reply 665–6.
24. Pieroni M, Dello Russo A, Marzo F, Pelargonio G, Casella M, Bellocci F, Crea F. High prevalence of myocarditis mimicking arrhythmogenic right ventricular cardiomyopathy differential diagnosis by electroanatomic mapping-guided endomyocardial biopsy. J Am Coll Cardiol. 2009;53:681–9.
25. Nery PB, Keren A, Healey J, Leug E, Beanlands RS, Birnie DH. Isolated cardiac sarcoidosis: establishing the diagnosis with electroanatomic mapping-guided endomyocardial biopsy. Can J Cardiol. 2013;29:1015.e1011–13.
26. Holzmann M, et al. Complication rate of right ventricular endomyocardial biopsy via the femoral approach. Circulation. 2008;118:1722–8.
27. Jang SY, et al. Complication rate of transfemoral endomyocardial biopsy with fluoroscopic and two-dimensional echocardiographic guidance: a 10-year experience of 228 consecutive procedures. J Korean Med Sci. 2013;28:1323–8.
28. Paul M, et al. Safety of endomyocardial biopsy in patients with arrhythmogenic right ventricular cardiomyopathy. JACC Cardiovasc Interv. 2011;4(10):1142–8.
29. Yilmaz A, et al. Comparative evaluation of left and right ventricular endomyocardial biopsy. Circulation. 2010;122:900–9.
30. Greif M. Cardiac sarcoidosis concealed by arrhythmogenic right ventricular dysplasia/cardiomyopathy. Nat Clin Pract Cardiovasc Med. 2008;5(4):231–6.

Chapter 9
Management of Arrhythmias Related to Cardiac Sarcoidosis

Matthew M. Zipse and William H. Sauer

Abstract Conduction disease in cardiac sarcoidosis is quite common and likely under-recognized. It also can be the first manifestation of the disease and deserves serious attention and a careful, comprehensive workup. Conduction disease can range from blocks at virtually all levels of the conduction system, and the development of both a wide variety of atrial and ventricular arrhythmias. There are several treatment strategies, and in appropriate patients, pharmacologic along with device therapy may be indicated.

Introduction

Because the initial presentation of cardiac sarcoidosis (CS) can range from asymptomatic electrocardiographic abnormalities to palpitations to sudden death, the cardiac electrophysiologist (EP) is an integral part of the multidisciplinary team taking care of sarcoidosis patients. Electrophysiologic findings, which often are under-recognized, are more common manifestations of CS than congestive heart failure (Table 9.1). Electrocardiography and invasive electrophysiologic testing are important components for the evaluation of cardiac sarcoidosis. After myocardial involvement has been established, patients with CS may meet an indication for implantable cardiac defibrillator implantation and require management of this device. This chapter will focus on cardiac arrhythmias and the cardiac electrophysiologist in the management of patients with sarcoidosis.

M.M. Zipse, MD • W.H. Sauer, MD (✉)
Section of Cardiac Electrophysiology, Division of Cardiology, University of Colorado Hospital, 12401 East 17th Avenue, B136, Aurora, CO 80045, USA
e-mail: Matthew.Zipse@ucdenver.edu; william.sauer@ucdenver.edu

© Springer International Publishing Switzerland 2015
A.M. Freeman, H.D. Weinberger (eds.), *Cardiac Sarcoidosis:*
Key Concepts in Pathogenesis, Disease Management, and Interesting Cases,
DOI 10.1007/978-3-319-14624-9_9

Table 9.1 Incident arrhythmic presentation of cardiac sarcoidosis [33]

	Prevalence in study series (%)
Atrioventricular block	26–67
Bundle branch block	12–61
Atrial arrhythmias	23–25
Ventricular arrhythmias	11–73
Sudden cardiac death	12–65
Congestive heart failure	10–30

Conduction System Disease

In cardiac sarcoidosis, granulomatous infiltration of the basal interventricular septum with resultant inflammation and subsequent scarring can cause injury to the various elements of the cardiac conduction system. This can result in a variety of conduction disturbances leading to bundle branch block or any level of atrioventricular block. Because of the progressive nature of CS, the level and severity of conduction block may also progress (Fig. 9.1).

Bundle Branch Block

Bundle branch block has been observed on surface electrocardiograms in 12–61 % of cases of CS, depending on study series [1–4]. Both the original and 2006 revised Japanese Ministry of Health and Welfare guidelines for the diagnosis of CS use RBBB as one of the ECG abnormalities constituting a minor diagnostic criterion [5]. While neither sensitive nor specific, both RBBB and LBBB are seen more commonly in patients with CS than those with sarcoidosis without myocardial involvement [4], and should prompt further investigations. Further studies are also needed to determine whether the presence of bundle branch block has prognostic implications for the future development of complete atrioventricular block or ventricular arrhythmias and sudden death in these patients.

Other Asymptomatic Electrocardiographic Findings

With inflammation and subsequent scarring in CS, areas of delayed myocardial activation are expected, and this can manifest as fragmentation on the surface ECG. While not included in previously-published diagnostic guidelines, QRS complex fragmentation, defined by the presence of an additional R wave (R′), notching in the nadir of the S wave, or the presence of >1 R′ in two anatomically contiguous leads (Fig. 9.2), was shown in two study series to carry more diagnostic value than RBBB alone [4, 6].

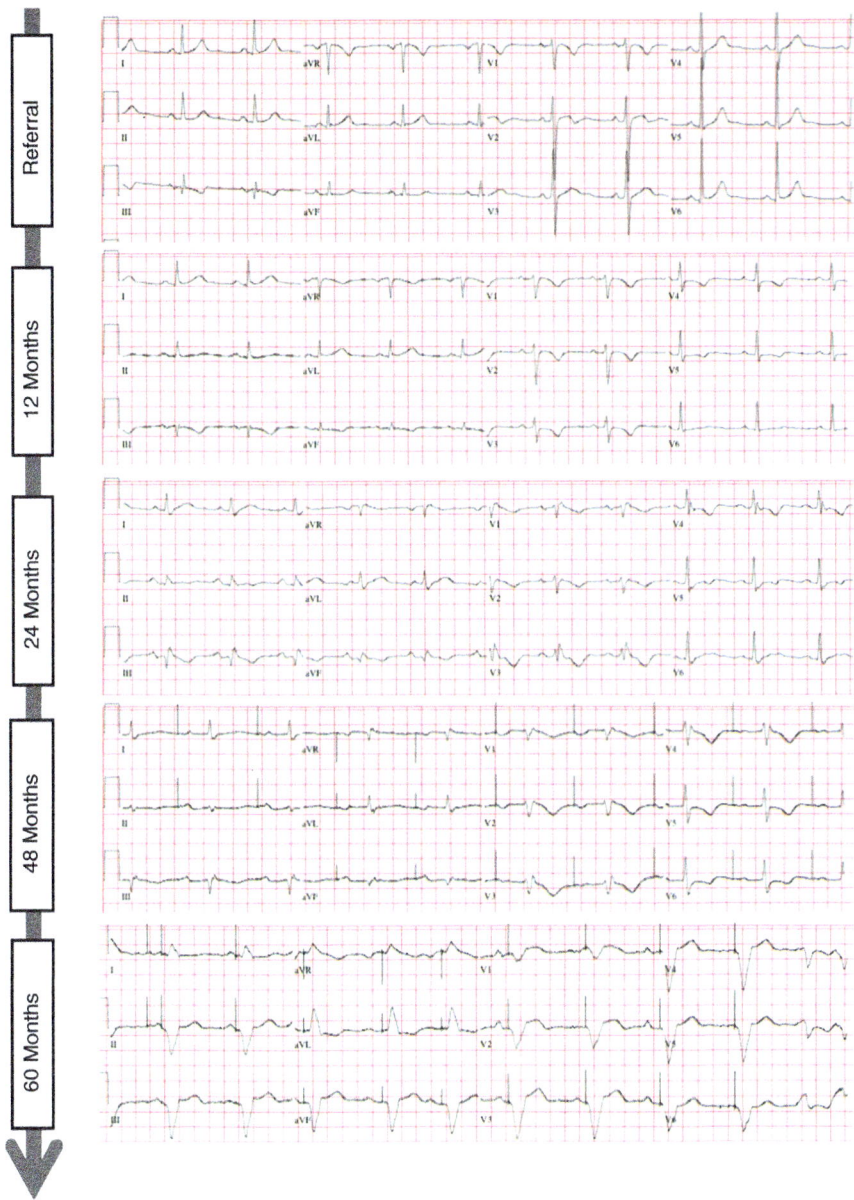

Fig. 9.1 Electrocardiographic progression of conduction system disease in a patient with cardiac sarcoidosis. Shown here is the progression (sequential ECGs, from *top*-to-*bottom*) in one patient over a period of 5 years from (*1*) sinus rhythm with a narrow QRS complex, to (*2*) first degree AV delay, to (*3*) RBBB, to (*4*) sinus node dysfunction with the need for atrial pacing, to (*5*) complete heart block with ventricular pacing

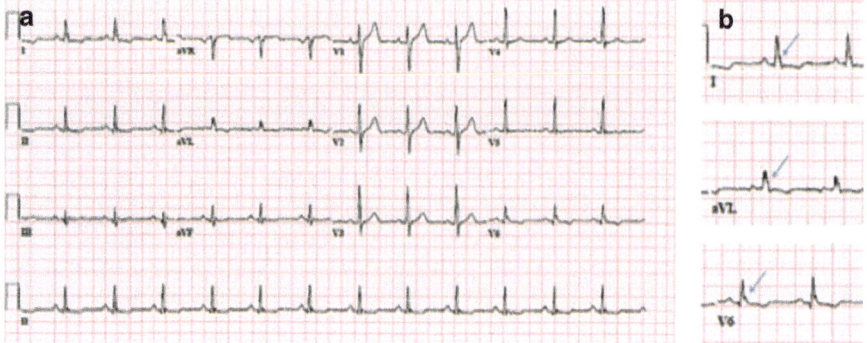

Fig. 9.2 ECG demonstrating QRS complex fragmentation and repolarization abnormalities (panel **a**), particularly notable in the lateral leads (*arrows*, panel **b**)

The signal-averaged ECG (SAECG) has utility in the detection of abnormal activation characterized by late potentials, and may also have both diagnostic and prognostic value [7]. Unlike the standard 12-lead ECG recording, requiring only a few seconds, SAECG recording requires up to 10 min, as multiple QRS potentials are averaged to allow both for the removal of interference due to skeletal muscle and for the detection of low amplitude, high frequency late potentials. While originally developed as a means of risk stratification in patients with coronary disease and cardiomyopathies to detect substrate for reentry, further investigations are needed to assess the abnormal SAECG as a risk marker for ventricular arrhythmias in CS.

Atrioventricular Block

Conduction block can range from first-degree atrioventricular delay to complete atrioventricular block, and the severity of block can progress with progression of inflammation and scar. Complete atrioventricular block (CAVB) is the one of the most common findings in patients with clinically-evident cardiac sarcoidosis, with a prevalence of 25 % in one retrospective analysis [1]. While usually felt to be related to infiltration of the conduction system itself, granulomatous involvement of the AV nodal artery has also been described as a cause of atrioventricular block in sarcoidosis [3]. CAVB often occurs at a younger age in patients with sarcoidosis than in individuals with complete heart block due to other etiologies.

Treatment of patients with high grade atrioventricular block with permanent pacing should be performed in accordance with published guidelines [8]. However, the presence of AV block likely signifies extensive myocardial involvement from sarcoidosis granuloma and portends a higher risk of future ventricular arrhythmias [9]. For this reason, the recently-published expert consensus statement from the Heart Rhythm Society related to the management of CS gives a Class IIa recommendation for ICD implantation (regardless of left ventricular ejection fraction) for the primary prevention of sudden cardiac death in CS if the patient meets an indication for pacing [10]. And, while there are no specific data related to the use of cardiac resynchronization therapy in CS patients, relevant recommendations based on major trials investigating biventricular pacing from the general device guidelines should apply to CS patients [8].

CAVB can be reversible in CS (see case vignette on recovery of atrioventricular conduction in Chap. 14), and there may be a role for immunosuppression in attempt to reverse CAVB. Kato et al. described their experience with 20 patients with CAVB and preserved left ventricular function [11]. AVB resolved in four of seven patients treated with corticosteroids (57 %), but did not improve in any of the untreated patients. In another study, atrioventricular conduction improved to normal in four of eight CAVB patients with relatively preserved left ventricular function, but in none of the four patients with advanced left ventricular dysfunction when given steroid treatment [12]. Accordingly, current guidelines state (with a Class IIa recommendation) that immunosuppression can be useful in CS patients with Mobitz II or third degree heart block.

Lastly, it should be noted that CAVB in young patients (less than 60 years of age) should prompt evaluation for sarcoidosis, even in those who do not carry a previous diagnosis of extracardiac sarcoidosis. CAVB can be the initial manifestation of cardiac involvement in patients with a prior diagnosis of systemic sarcoidosis, as well as the first clinical manifestation of sarcoidosis from any organ. This was the case in a Japanese study of 89 consecutive patients with no known history of sarcoidosis with high-grade atrioventricular block requiring permanent dual chamber pacemaker implantation that were prospectively evaluated for cardiac sarcoidosis. Ten cases (11.2 %) of cardiac sarcoidosis were diagnosed, most frequently in young women aged 40–69 (32 %) [13]. Kandolin et al. investigated 72 patients (age <55 years) with unexplained AV block and found biopsy-verified CS in 14 (19 %) and 'probable' CS in 4 (6 %) of the 72 patients [14]. Patients with sarcoidosis had a significantly more adverse prognosis when compared to patients with idiopathic AV block in this series.

Sinus Node Dysfunction

Extensive granulatomous lesions in the sinoatrial node subendocardium have previously been described in autopsy series [15, 16], and sinus node dysfunction may be an under-recognized manifestation of CS [17]. Figure 9.3 shows an electrocardiogram of a patient with sinus node dysfunction and CS, ultimately leading to sinus arrest, and ultimately a polymorphic VT arrest. Patients with sinus node dysfunction may have an indication for permanent pacing, and if this is the case, dual chamber ICD implantation may be reasonable.

Atrial Arrhythmias

Supraventricular arrhythmias and atrial fibrillation are common in CS, with a prevalence ranging from 23 to 36 % (Fig. 9.4) [18–20]. In a study of 100 consecutive patients with biopsy-proven systemic sarcoidosis and evidence of cardiac

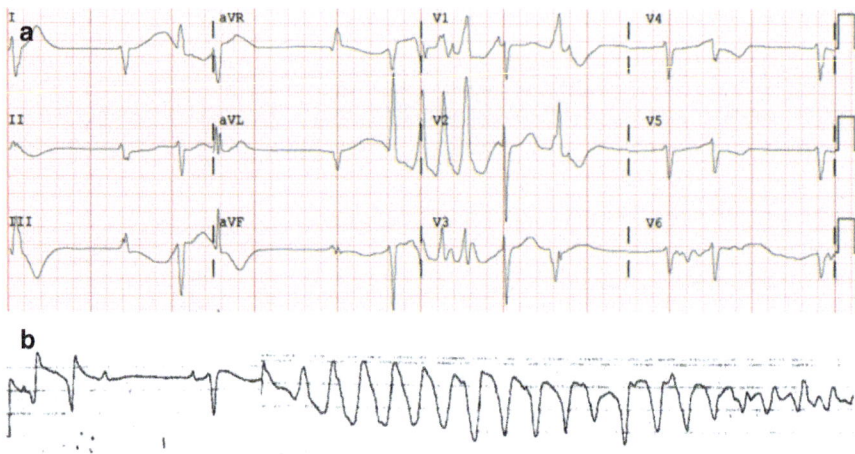

Fig. 9.3 A 12-lead ECG in a patient with CS showing sinus arrest, inferior QRS fragmentation, and QT prolongation with EADs (**a**), ultimately leading to a polymorphic VT arrest (**b**)

involvement by MRI, PET, or endomyocardial biopsy, a 32 % prevalence of supraventricular arrhythmias was observed over a mean follow-up period of 5.8 years. Arrhythmias were documented by ECG, device interrogation data, or ambulatory telemetry monitoring. Atrial fibrillation was the most common supraventricular arrhythmia reported, accounting for 56 % of those described. After multivariate analysis, left-atrial enlargement was the only parameter significantly associated with supraventricular arrhythmias (HR 6.12, 2.2–17.1, P<0.01) [18].

A similar prevalence of atrial arrhythmias was described in a separate retrospective series, in which 16/44 (36 %) patients with evidence of CS by cardiac magnetic resonance imaging (CMR) had documented atrial arrhythmias, the most common of which was atrial tachycardia (18 %). In the 26 patients with ICDs in this cohort, 11.5 % received inappropriate ICD therapies for atrial arrhythmias [20]. This was similar to the 12 % incidence of inappropriate therapies in a separate study [21].

Atrial arrhythmias arise from a variety of mechanisms in CS. In a third recently-investigated series, 15/65 patients (23 %) with CS experienced 28 distinct symptomatic supraventricular arrhythmias (9 Atrial Fibrillation; 3 Atrial Flutter; 16 Atrial Tachycardia). These patients ultimately underwent electrophysiologic testing to characterize the arrhythmias. The mechanism of atrial arrhythmias was determined to be from triggered activity in 11 %, abnormal automaticity in 47 %, and reentrant in 42 % of the non-AF atrial arrhythmias. Inflammation and edema associated with the initial infiltrative stage and scar that manifests as the disease progresses to the fibrotic stage likely independently account for the differing mechanisms observed.

The variety of mechanisms and differing substrate for atrial arrhythmias in CS suggests that management of atrial arrhythmias may require a multi-faceted approach including immunosuppression, antiarrhythmic therapy, catheter ablation, or a combination of these strategies for arrhythmia control. Immunosuppression is

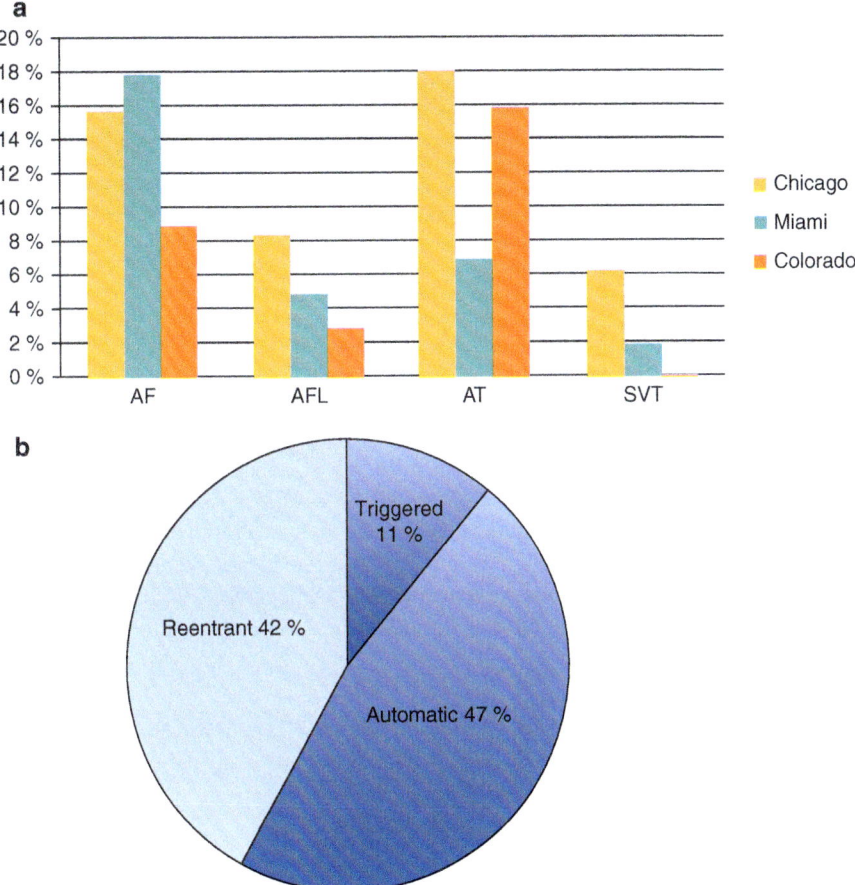

Fig. 9.4 The prevalence of atrial arrhythmias are shown here (**a**) from three different cohorts of CS patients from studies at the University of Chicago [20], University of Miami [18], and University of Colorado [19]. The mechanisms of atrial arrhythmias in CS are diverse (**b**) [19]

discussed in greater detail in subsequent chapters, though the three study series described above each employed immunosuppression with variable results. In one of the series, the overall burden of atrial fibrillation appeared to decrease with immunosuppression [19]. Anti-arrhythmic therapy might include the use of class IC agents, class III agents, or beta-blockers. The efficacy of these drugs for the control of atrial arrhythmias has not been specifically studied in CS.

Lastly, catheter ablation appears to be tolerated and efficacious in patients with CS. In a recent study reporting on a local experience of catheter ablation of atrial arrhythmias in nine CS patients with ten different atrial arrhythmias, two patients had recurrences requiring repeat procedures, but all ultimately became arrhythmia free over a limited 1.8 year mean follow-up period. There were no complications reported in this small case series [22].

Ventricular Arrhythmias

Just as atrial inflammation and fibrosis can lead to atrial arrhythmias in CS, involvement of the ventricular myocardium can lead to ventricular arrhythmias (Fig. 9.5) by similar triggered, automatic, and reentrant mechanisms [23–27]. Prior to the use of the implanted cardiac defibrillator (ICD), sudden death secondary to ventricular tachyarrhythmias accounted for approximately 25–65 % of deaths caused by CS [2, 3, 28]. Furthermore, ventricular arrhythmias have frequently been described as the initial presentation of CS [29]. In patients with CS, an ICD may be indicated, and this is discussed in detail in Chap. 12.

Inflammation associated with granuloma infiltration can play a significant role in the exacerbation of electrical storm in CS patients. Schuller et al. found the incidence of *ICD storm*, defined as three or more appropriate ICD therapies in 24 h, to be particularly high – 11 % (16 of 112 patients) in their cohort [21]. Predictors of ICD storm included left ventricular dysfunction (OR 6.71 [95 % CI 1.45–31.2], P=0.015) and right ventricular dysfunction (OR 3.86 [95 % CI 1.16–12.8], P=0.03), suggesting that more extensive myocardial involvement is a predisposing factor to electrical storm.

Because corticosteroids can play an integral role in arrhythmia suppression, treatment in new presentations with ventricular tachycardia (VT) or ventricular fibrillation (VF) should begin with assessment for active inflammatory sarcoidosis

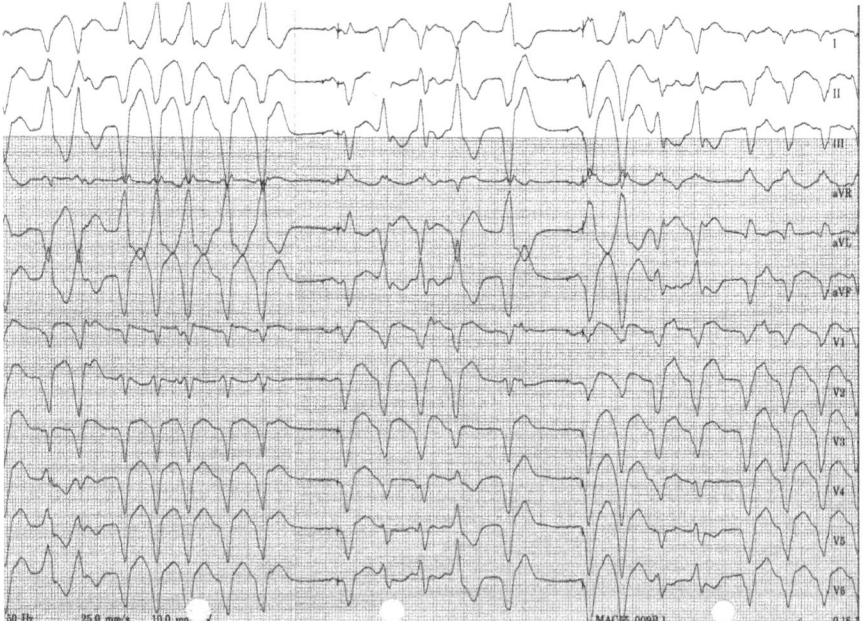

Fig. 9.5 A case of spontaneous pleomorphic ventricular tachycardia in a patient with cardiac sarcoidosis (Courtesy of Fermin Garcia, MD)

myocarditis and therapy with immunosuppression as indicated [25, 30, 31]. In other cases of VT in cardiac sarcoidosis, the disease has already progressed to the fibrotic stage and generated scar. As in patients with other cardiomyopathies and VT, scar serves as substrate for reentry by creating both a zone of slow conduction and an anatomical barrier around which a circuit may propagate [27].

Ventricular arrhythmias in sarcoidosis patients, when present, can be more difficult to control (both with anti-arrhythmic therapy and by catheter ablation) than in patients with other cardiomyopathies because ventricular involvement is frequently more diffuse and heterogeneous. The complicated pattern of scarring that occurs with CS can provide substrate for circuits involving the endocardium, epicardium, and mid-myocardium.

Anti-arrhythmic Drugs for Ventricular Arrhythmias

Corticosteroids alone can be ineffective at preventing monomorphic VT [23, 25, 26], as disease progression through the inflammatory stage has sometimes already progressed to scar formation creating an arrhythmic substrate, which is unlikely to be reversed with immunosuppression. Anti-arrhythmic drug use varies widely and can include beta blockers, Class IA, IB, IC, and III agents – used both in isolation or in combination, each with variable outcome [25, 27, 32, 33]. Mohsen et al. reported that of the 21 patients in their series requiring anti-arrhythmic drugs, nine patients continued to have ventricular arrhythmias and appropriate ICD therapies (with a mean of 8.7 shocks per patient over a mean 4-year follow-up period).

Catheter Ablation of Ventricular Arrhythmias

Medical therapy alone is commonly ineffective at complete arrhythmia suppression [23], in which case catheter ablation may be indicated. Jefic et al. have reported on nine patients with CS and VT who underwent radiofrequency ablation, resulting in elimination of 31 of 44 (70 %) inducible VTs, and a subsequent decrease (n=4) or complete elimination (n=5) of VT over a mean follow-up period of 20 months [25]. Most of the VTs were re-entrant in mechanism, and VTs were found to be both endocardial and epicardial in origin, as well as left- and right-sided, though the most prevalent location of reentry (7/21 VTs) was the tricuspid annulus.

Koplan et al. reported their experience of VT ablation in CS patients, with contrasting results to Jefic et al. In their case series, half of the patients were referred for heart transplantation for recurrent VTs post-ablation, and most patients (6/8) had recurrent VT [24]. In this series, patients tended to have more severe left ventricular dysfunction, suggesting that arrhythmic substrate in the former series may have been more localized and amenable to radiofrequency ablation. Ultimately, with the varied severity of disease burden, a combination approach including immunosuppression, anti-arrhythmic therapy, and catheter ablation may be required for arrhythmia control in CS.

Conclusion

Cardiac sarcoidosis can present in the setting of advanced systemic disease or in clinical isolation. The manifestations of CS are highly variable: myocardial involvement can be subclinical, or it may lead to atrioventricular block, heart failure, atrial and ventricular arrhythmias, or sudden cardiac death.

Conduction system disease, either symptomatic or asymptomatic, is the most common presentation of CS. Young patients presenting with heart block may have underlying sarcoidosis; accordingly, all patients under the age of 60 presenting with idiopathic heart block should be screened for CS. Among patients with CS, pacing is indicated for higher levels of heart block, but the presence of heart block is an independent predictor of appropriate ICD therapy and therefore consideration of dual chamber ICD or CRT-D implantation should be given if sarcoidosis is known to be the cause of the heart block.

Ventricular arrhythmias are the second most common presentation of cardiac sarcoidosis. These arise when sarcoidosis granulomas within the myocardium lead to inflammation or scar and become foci for abnormal automaticity, triggered activity, or reentry. Management of ventricular arrhythmias often requires a combination of immunosuppression, anti-arrhythmic therapy, and catheter ablation.

In addition to conduction disease and ventricular arrhythmias, other described arrhythmias include ectopic atrial activity, paroxysmal atrial tachycardia, atrial flutter, atrial fibrillation, and sinus arrest secondary to granulomatous involvement of the sinus node. These atrial arrhythmias arise from diverse mechanisms, and may also be amenable to anti-arrhythmic therapy and catheter ablation.

Pearls of Wisdom
1. Cardiac sarcoidosis can present in the setting of advanced systemic disease or in clinical isolation.
2. The manifestations of CS are highly variable: myocardial involvement can be subclinical, or it may lead to atrioventricular block, heart failure, atrial and ventricular arrhythmias, or sudden cardiac death.
3. All patients under the age of 60 presenting with idiopathic heart block should be screened for CS.
4. Ventricular arrhythmias are the second most common presentation of cardiac sarcoidosis. These arise when sarcoidosis granulomas within the myocardium lead to inflammation or scar and become foci for abnormal automaticity, triggered activity, or reentry. Management of ventricular arrhythmias often requires a combination of immunosuppression, anti-arrhythmic therapy, catheter ablation, and implantable cardioverter-defibrillators.
5. Because the overall burden of arrhythmia and conduction disease is high in patients with CS and management is complex and multifaceted, the cardiac electrophysiologist plays an important role in the multidisciplinary care of these patients.

Because the overall burden of arrhythmia and conduction disease is high in patients with CS and management is complex and multifaceted, the cardiac electrophysiologist plays an important role in the multidisciplinary care of these patients.

References

1. Chapelon-Abric C, de Zuttere D, Duhaut P, Veyssier P, Wechsler B, Huong DLT, et al. Cardiac sarcoidosis. Medicine. 2004;83:315–34.
2. Matsui Y, Iwai K, Tachibana T, Fruie T, Shigematsu N, Izumi T, et al. Clinicopathological study of fatal myocardial sarcoidosis. Ann N Y Acad Sci. 1976;278:455–69.
3. Roberts WC, McAllister HA, Ferrans VJ. Sarcoidosis of the heart. A clinicopathologic study of 35 necropsy patients (group 1) and review of 78 previously described necropsy patients (group 11). Am J Med. 1977;63:86–108.
4. Schuller JL, Olson MD, Zipse MM, Schneider PM, Aleong RG, Weinberger HD, et al. Electrocardiographic characteristics in patients with pulmonary sarcoidosis indicating cardiac involvement. J Cardiovasc Electrophysiol. 2011;22:1243–8.
5. Soejima K, Yada H. The work-up and management of patients with apparent or subclinical cardiac sarcoidosis: with emphasis on the associated heart rhythm abnormalities. J Cardiovasc Electrophysiol. 2009;20:578–83. Wiley Online Library.
6. Homsi M, Alsayed L, Safadi B, Mahenthiran J, Das MK. Fragmented QRS complexes on 12-lead ECG: a marker of cardiac sarcoidosis as detected by gadolinium cardiac magnetic resonance imaging. Ann Noninvasive Electrocardiol. 2009;14:319–26.
7. Schuller JL, Lowery CM, Zipse M, Aleong RG, Varosy PD, Weinberger HD, et al. Diagnostic utility of signal-averaged electrocardiography for detection of cardiac sarcoidosis. Ann Noninvasive Electrocardiol. 2011;16:70–6.
8. Epstein AE, DiMarco JP, Ellenbogen KA, Estes NAM, Freedman RA, Gettes LS, et al. ACCF/AHA/HRS focused update incorporated into the ACCF/AHA/HRS 2008 guidelines for device-based therapy of cardiac rhythm abnormalities: a report of the American College of Cardiology Foundation/American Heart Association Task Force on Practice Guidelines and the Heart Rhythm Society. Circulation. 2012;2013:e283–352.
9. Betensky BP, Tschabrunn CM, Zado ES, Goldberg LR, Marchlinski FE, Garcia FC, et al. Long-term follow-up of patients with cardiac sarcoidosis and implantable cardioverter-defibrillators. HRTHM. 2012;9:884–91. Elsevier Inc.
10. Birnie DH, Sauer W, Bogun F, Cooper J, Culver DA, Duvernoy C, et al. Heart rhythm society expert consensus statement on the diagnosis and management of arrhythmias associated with cardiac sarcoidosis. HRTHM. 2014;11(7):1304–1323. Elsevier (In Press).
11. Kato Y, Morimoto S-I, Uemura A, Hiramitsu S, Ito T, Hishida H. Efficacy of corticosteroids in sarcoidosis presenting with atrioventricular block. Sarcoidosis Vasc Diffuse Lung Dis. 2003;20:133–7.
12. Yodogawa K, Seino Y, Ohara T, Takayama H, Katoh T, Mizuno K. Effect of corticosteroid therapy on ventricular arrhythmias in patients with cardiac sarcoidosis. Ann Noninvasive Electrocardiol. 2011;16:140–7.
13. Yoshida Y, Morimoto S, Hiramitsu S, Tsuboi N, Hirayama H, Itoh T. Incidence of cardiac sarcoidosis in Japanese patients with high-degree atrioventricular block. Am Heart J. 1997;134:382–6.
14. Kandolin R, Lehtonen J, Kupari M. Cardiac sarcoidosis and giant cell myocarditis as causes of atrioventricular block in young and middle-aged adults. Circ Arrhythm Electrophysiol. 2011;4:303–9.
15. Gozo EG, Cosnow I, Cohen HC, Okun L. The heart in sarcoidosis. Chest. 1971;60:379–88. American College of Chest Physicians.
16. Abeler V. Sarcoidosis of the cardiac conducting system. Am Heart J. 1979;97:701–7.

17. Ton K, Schulman S, Lima J, Tandri H. Cardiac sarcoidosis presenting as sick sinus syndrome and recurrent ventricular tachycardia. HRS Journal of the American College of Cardiology 2014;63(125):1–1.
18. Viles-Gonzalez JF, Pastori L, Fischer A, Wisnivesky JP, Goldman MG, Mehta D. Supraventricular arrhythmias in patients with cardiac sarcoidosis: prevalence, predictors and clinical implications. Chest. 2013;143:1085–90.
19. Zipse MM, Schuller JL, Katz DF, Steckman DA, Gonzalez JE, Sung RK, et al. Atrial arrhythmias are common and arise from diverse mechanisms in patients with cardiac sarcoidosis. Heart Rhythm 2013;10(S309):1–2.
20. Cain MA, Metzl MD, Patel AR, Addetia K. Cardiac sarcoidosis detected by Late Gadolinium enhancement and prevalence of atrial arrhythmias. Am J Cardiol. 2014;113:1556–60.
21. Schuller JL, Zipse M, Crawford T, Bogun F, Beshai J, Patel AR, et al. Implantable cardioverter defibrillator therapy in patients with cardiac sarcoidosis. J Cardiovasc Electrophysiol. 2012;23:925–9.
22. Willner JM, Viles-Gonzalez JF, Coffey JO, Morgenthau A, Mehta D. Catheter ablation of atrial arrhythmias in cardiac sarcoidosis. J Cardiovasc Electrophysiol. 2014;25:958–63.
23. Winters SL, Cohen M, Greenberg S, Stein B, Curwin J, Pe E, et al. Sustained ventricular tachycardia associated with sarcoidosis: assessment of the underlying cardiac anatomy and the prospective utility of programmed ventricular stimulation, drug therapy and an implantable antitachycardia device. JAC. 1991;18:937–43.
24. Koplan BA, Soejima K, Baughman K, Epstein LM, Stevenson WG. Refractory ventricular tachycardia secondary to cardiac sarcoid: electrophysiologic characteristics, mapping, and ablation. HRTHM. 2006;3:924–9.
25. Jefic D, Joel B, Good E, Morady F, Rosman H, Knight B, et al. Role of radiofrequency catheter ablation of ventricular tachycardia in cardiac sarcoidosis: report from a multicenter registry. Heart Rhythm. 2009;6:189–95.
26. Banba K, Kusano KF, Nakamura K, Morita H, Ogawa A, Ohtsuka F, et al. Relationship between arrhythmogenesis and disease activity in cardiac sarcoidosis. HRTHM. 2007;4:1292–9.
27. Furushima H, Chinushi M, Sugiura H, Kasai H, Washizuka T, Aizawa Y. Ventricular tachyarrhythmia associated with cardiac sarcoidosis: its mechanisms and outcome. Clin Cardiol. 2004;27:217–22.
28. Fleming HA, Bailey SM. Sarcoid heart disease. J R Coll Physicians Lond. 1981;15:245.
29. Uusimaa P, Ylitalo K, Anttonen O, Kerola T, Virtanen V, Pääkkö E, et al. Ventricular tachyarrhythmia as a primary presentation of sarcoidosis. Europace. 2008;10:760–6.
30. Stees CS, Khoo MSC, Lowery CM, Sauer WH. Ventricular tachycardia storm successfully treated with immunosuppression and catheter ablation in a patient with cardiac sarcoidosis. J Cardiovasc Electrophysiol. 2011;22:210–3.
31. Yazaki Y, Isobe M, Hiroe M, Morimoto S-I, Hiramitsu S, Nakano T, et al. Prognostic determinants of long-term survival in Japanese patients with cardiac sarcoidosis treated with prednisone. Am J Cardiol. 2001;88:1006–10. Elsevier.
32. Mohsen A, Jimenez A, Hood RE, Dickfeld T, Saliaris A, Shorofsky S, et al. Cardiac sarcoidosis: electrophysiological outcomes on long-term follow-up and the role of the implantable cardioverter-defibrillator. J Cardiovasc Electrophysiol. 2014;25(2):171–76.
33. Zipse MM, Sauer WH. Electrophysiologic manifestations of cardiac sarcoidosis. Curr Opin Pulm Med. 2013;19:485–92.

Chapter 10
Acute Management of Cardiac Sarcoidosis

Neal K. Lakdawala and Garrick C. Stewart

Abstract The initial presentation of cardiac sarcoidosis (CS) may be in the acute care setting with heart block, ventricular tachycardia (VT) or acute heart failure (HF). Cardiovascular clinicians should consider sarcoidosis in the differential diagnosis when confronting these relatively common problems, especially where the patient is relatively young and once coronary heart disease has been excluded. Corticosteroids are the principal immunosuppressant used in the acute setting, owing to its relatively rapid effect. Although minimal controlled data are available to guide the use of corticosteroids, they have been most effective in resolving AV block. Accordingly, conventional management of VT and HF should be also be utilized.

Introduction

Clinicians encountering cardiac sarcoidosis (CS) in an acute care setting are charged with managing a potentially life threatening disease without the benefit of a robust database of clinical trials on which to base their management. Accordingly, this chapter reflects one group's approach to this disease based upon the limited information available in the medical literature and enhanced by clinical experience. Hopefully this is a salvo in a sustained effort to improve our collective abilities to diagnose, risk stratify and manage patients with this vexing illness.

One key factor in managing acute presentations of CS is *recognizing* the disease. Indeed there are several practical reasons to include CS in the differential diagnosis of atrioventricular (AV) block, ventricular tachycardia (VT) and acute heart failure with systolic dysfunction. For one, anti-inflammatory therapies are generally considered more effective if initiated prior to end-stage disease. Second, diagnosis of CS may influence device utilization in the setting of conduction disease. As reviewed in Chap. 12 and elsewhere, the general practice is to implant a cardioverter

---

N.K. Lakdawala, MD (✉) • G.C. Stewart, MD
Cardiovascular Medicine, Brigham and Women's Hospital, Harvard Medical School, 75 Francis Street, Boston, MA, USA
e-mail: NLAKDAWALA@PARTNERS.ORG; gcstewart@partners.org

defibrillator (ICD) in lieu of a pacemaker (PPM) [1]. Moreover, a CS diagnosis may be unnecessarily delayed by conventional management of heart rhythm disorders. For example, PPM or ICD implantation typically precludes future cardiac magnetic resonance imaging (CMR) and delays endomyocardial biopsy as newly placed leads could by displaced by the bioptome. Moreover, radiofrequency ablation may confound the use of ^{18}F-labeled fluorodeoxyglucose (FDG) positron emission tomography (PET) to identify cardiac inflammation.

When to Suspect Cardiac Sarcoidosis

Infrahissian AV block (either Mobitz II or 3rd degree), monomorphic VT (often multifocal) and heart failure with reduced left ventricular systolic function are the principle cardiac manifestations of sarcoidosis which can culminate in presentation to an acute care setting. Associated symptoms include syncope, cardiac arrest, dyspnea, and reduced exercise capacity. Much less commonly an acute presentation of CS is secondary to mitral regurgitation or pericardial effusion.

Heart failure and arrhythmia are amongst the most common general reasons for cardiac hospitalization. How then to recognize a rare cause (sarcoidosis) hidden amongst the many presentations of ischemic and hypertensive heart disease? The approach below is to consider different scenarios, where the pre-test probability of CS ranges from relatively high (cardiac presentation in patients with known systemic sarcoidosis) to low (index presentation of isolated CS). In each of these different scenarios, alternate diagnoses should be considered, especially ischemic heart disease, which by virtue of its high prevalence, is a likely cause of cardiac hospitalization regardless of the pretest probability for CS.

Cardiac Manifestations in Patients with Known Systemic Sarcoidosis

Patients presenting with acute cardiac manifestations of sarcoidosis in the context of an established diagnosis of systemic sarcoidosis should be readily recognized by providers. Different diagnostic criteria can be used in this setting (Table 10.1). These tools are expert consensus documents that have not been empirically derived nor well validated. The Japanese Ministry of Health and Welfare (JMHW) criteria were first established in 1993 [2] and refined in 2007 [1]. Definite diagnosis of CS according to the JMHW criteria are present if a noncaseating granuloma is seen in the myocardium – or – probable diagnosis of CS is made if a patient with proven extra cardiac sarcoidosis has a combination of electrocardiographic findings plus either abnormal cardiac imaging or hemodynamics. The Heart Rhythm Society (HRS) and the World Association of Sarcoidosis and Other Granulomatous (WASOG) disorders have recently provided similar consensus recommendations

Table 10.1 Consensus diagnostic criteria for cardiac sarcoidosis

	JMHW	HRS 2014
Definite diagnosis	Histologic evidence of cardiac non-caseating granuloma	Histologic evidence of cardiac non-caseating granuloma, with no alternative cause identified (i.e., infection)
Probable/clinical diagnosis	Histological diagnosis of extra-cardiac sarcoidosis **And** ECG abnormalities: right bundle branch block, left axis deviation, VT, premature ventricular contractions, ST-T wave abnormalities or Q wave **And** one of the following: 1. Echocardiographic evidence of regional wall motion abnormalities or left ventricular dilation 2. Nuclear imaging: perfusion defect or cardiac Gallium/PYP uptake 3. Invasive hemodynamics: increased ventricular filling pressures, reduced cardiac output 4. Biopsy: interstitial fibrosis or cellular infiltration	Histological diagnosis of extra-cardiac sarcoidosis **And** one or more of the following: 1. Steroid/immunosuppressant responsive cardiomyopathy or AV block 2. Unexplained reduced LVEF (<40 %) 3. Unexplained sustained VT (spontaneous or induced) 4. Mobitz type II or 3rd degree AV block 5. Patchy uptake on dedicated cardiac PET[a] 6. Late gadolinium enhancement on CMR[a] 7. Positive gallium uptake[a] **And** other causes for cardiac manifestations have been reasonably excluded

CMR cardiac magnetic resonance imaging, *PET* positron emission tomography, *JMHW* Japanese Ministry of Health and Welfare criteria, *VT* ventricular tachycardia
[a]In a pattern consistent with cardiac sarcoidosis

for the diagnosis of cardiac sarcoidosis. Like the JHMW criteria, definite CS diagnosis can be made if microscopic examination of the heart reveals noncaseating granulomas – or – probable diagnosis can be made in the context of pathologically confirmed systemic disease and non-invasive evidence of cardiac abnormalities [1, 3].

Cardiac Manifestations in Patents with Hitherto Unknown Systemic Sarcoidosis

Although there is a broad differential diagnosis for the presenting symptoms of CS, in young patients without ischemic heart disease, the likelihood of underlying CS increases. Accordingly, patients without previously known systemic sarcoidosis should be queried for history suggestive of multisystem involvement (e.g. cough, iritis, dermatologic abnormalities). Here, the identification of non-cardiac involvement and establishment of diagnosis through histologic evaluation (e.g. lymph node biopsy) can be pivotal.

Cardiac Manifestations in Patients with Isolated Cardiac Sarcoidosis

The diagnosis of sarcoidosis limited to the heart without extra-cardiac features is challenging. The classic teaching is that isolated CS is rare, however the epidemiologic data are suspect. Anecdotal experience includes patients only recognized to have CS at the time of cardiac transplantation, when the explant is carefully examined by a pathologist, or at autopsy. Our general approach is to extensively evaluate for CS in young patients presenting with infrahissian block, dilated cardiomyopathy with conduction disease and/or arrhythmia, or repetitive multifocal monomorphic VT.

A relatively high prevalence of CS has been reported in adult patients younger than 60 presenting with AV block [4]. In a single center prospective study utilizing FDG-PET in 32 young and middle aged adults presenting with idiopathic AV block, CS was identified in 34 % of subjects. All were subsequently found to have systemic sarcoidosis. In addition to ischemic heart disease, Lyme carditis and inherited neuromuscular disease should be considered alongside CS in these patients.

In patients without ischemic heart disease who present with sustained VT, cardiac sarcoidosis may be present in up to 10 % of cases [5, 6]. These patients are usually middle aged with multifocal monomorphic VT and electrophysiological evidence of scar reentry. Left ventricular systolic dysfunction and AV block often, but not universally, coexist with VT in these patients.

Dilated cardiomyopathy with conduction disease and/or arrhythmia (DCM+E) has been variably described in the literature as conduction cardiomyopathy [7], DCM+E [8] or arrhythmogenic cardiomyopathy [9]. By recognizing a heavy burden of conduction disease and/or arrhythmia in DCM, the differential diagnosis can be narrowed to a number of etiologies with specific therapeutic and prognostic implications [8]. Broadly categorized, DCM+E can be caused by ischemic, genetic, infections, and inflammatory etiologies. Once ischemic heart disease has been excluded, key clinical features can be used to distinguish amongst the other pathologies and definitive testing is often available.

A family history of unexplained sudden death, heart failure or cardiac transplantation should be obtained. Genetic testing, inclusive of genes commonly mutated in DCM+E (LMNA, DES, SCN5A, EMD, DSP, PKP2, DSC2), is now widely available. Although results will not be available for up to 14 weeks, the identification of a disease causing DNA variant in the appropriate clinical context can provide definitive diagnostic information allowing the reasonable exclusion of alternate etiologies including CS along with the identification of at risk family members [10, 11].

Residence or extended travel to areas where infection with Trypanosoma cruzi is endemic is key to identifying patients with Chagas heart disease [12]. Like CS, Chagas heart disease can present with conduction disease, regional wall motion abnormalities and ventricular tachyarrhythmia. Serologic testing in the appropriate setting can identify patients with Chagas heart disease and can enable therapy with anti-parasitic therapies such as benznidazole which may alter the natural history of this otherwise unrelenting disease [13]. Moreover, erroneous use of immunosuppression for presumed CS in a patient with Chagas heart disease could lead to accelerated pathogenesis [14].

Giant cell myocarditis (GCM) is a rare but devastating inflammatory cardiomyopathy with many of the same clinical features of CS, albeit with a rapidly progressive course. Amongst patients presenting with rapidly progressive cardiomyopathy, often without dilated remodeling, GCM should be considered. Although therapy for giant cell myocarditis is unrefined, its identification should prompt consideration for cardiac transplantation owing to its generally poor prognosis. Unlike CS where the yield of endomyocardial biopsy is generally low (see Chap. 9) the diffuse myocardial involvement in GCM is usually readily apparent on biopsy.

Acute Evaluations for Cardiac Sarcoidosis

Our approach to the evaluation of sarcoidosis is context dependent, as enumerated above. In patients with proven systemic disease, the exclusion of coronary heart disease and either FDG-PET or CMR findings suggestive of CS are usually sufficient to make a diagnosis. However, we prioritize this testing to precede ICD implantation or radiofrequency ablation due to the limiting/confounding effects of these therapies on non-invasive testing. Amongst patients with suspected isolated CS, we perform a thorough evaluation for extra-cardiac sarcoidosis, enhanced with FDG-PET. If not present, we have a low threshold to perform endomyocardial biopsy. In this setting, the performance of voltage guided biopsy may increase the diagnostic yield and is generally favored [15, 16]. As noted earlier, the implantation of a PPM or ICD usually limits the performance of biopsy for at least a month due to concerns of lead dislodgement.

Acute Medical Management of Cardiac Sarcoidosis

Medical therapy initiated in the acute care setting should be undertaken based on the severity of cardiac involvement and with a broader perspective of the patient's multisystem involvement, prior therapies, and clinical trajectory. The response to prior immunosuppressive therapy, including corticosteroids and the use of steroid sparing agents is an important consideration. The presence of severe extra-cardiac disease may justify immunosuppressive therapy ipso facto. To the contrary, patients with advanced or end-stage cardiac involvement may have little to gain from immunosuppression and may only suffer its adverse consequences.

The content below focuses on the use of corticosteroid immunosuppression and presupposes that conventional therapies for heart failure (diuretics, neuro-hormonal antagonists) and arrhythmia (antiarrhythmic drugs, radiofrequency ablation) are used. In general, a diagnosis of CS should lead to the addition of immunosuppressive medications on top of conventional therapies.

As described in detail in Chap. 11, immunosuppressive therapies are frequently utilized in CS, albeit without prospective or well-designed clinical studies to inform dose, duration or extent of efficacy. The published studies likely reflect some degree of publication and ascertainment bias and usually only describe an individual center's approach to management. Indeed the limitations of the published literature were highlighted in a recently published systemic review of the literature by Nery and colleagues [17]. They concluded that the best data exist for the efficacy of steroids for the management of AV block related to sarcoidosis and that the existing literature pertaining to VT and heart failure do not enable a statement of efficacy.

Of the different immunosuppressive agents used in sarcoidosis, the experience is greatest with corticosteroids. Because corticosteroids have a rapid onset of action, they are generally the agent used in the acute setting where rapid control of inflammation is desired. Steroid sparing agents such as methotrexate typically require weeks to take effect and accordingly are not reviewed here.

Our general approach to corticosteroid therapy is to initiate prednisone at high dose (0.5 mg/kg), which is then gradually tapered off over the ensuing 6–12 months. The use of non-invasive imaging and clinical cues to guide the weaning of steroids is detailed elsewhere in this text. However, prior to the initiation of high dose corticosteroids for CS, providers are advised to assess for risk of complications and prepare the patient accordingly (Table 10.2). This includes a test for latent tuberculosis infection and subsequent management, as well as an assessment for osteoporosis and glucose intolerance.

Scenarios Where Corticosteroids May Be Useful in the Acute Management of Cardiac Sarcoidosis

Atrioventricular Block

The best data in support of corticosteroid therapy for CS are for patients presenting with AV block. As summarized by Sadek and colleagues [17], 6 studies, including a total of 73 patients, have reported the outcomes associated with steroid therapy in patients presenting AV block. Amongst 57 patients treated with steroids, nearly half had resolution of AV block, whereas recovery of conduction occurred in none of the 16 patients not receiving steroids. As noted previously, ICD implantation in lieu of a standard dual chamber pacemaker should be strongly considered in patients requiring pacing for symptomatic conduction disease [1].

Ventricular Tachycardia

There are extremely limited data to inform the use of corticosteroids to manage symptomatic VT in CS. As the underlying etiology appears to be related to scar reentry [5], and reduction in inflammation is not expected to reduce scar burden,

Table 10.2 Testing and management for selected corticosteroid therapy toxicities

Corticosteroid toxicities	Pre-initiation testing	Management
Activation of latent tuberculosis	Test for latent TB infection (purified protein derivative, interferon-gamma release assay)	Treatment of latent TB
Opportunistic infection (e.g. pneumocystis)	HIV	Consider prophylaxis in selected patients with trimethoprim/sulfamethoxazole or alternative
Hypertension	Blood pressure	Hypertension management
Weight gain	Body mass index	Dietician consult
Glucose intolerance	Fasting glucose, glycosylated hemoglobin concentration (Hgb A1C)	Serial measurement of fasting glucose
		Medical therapy
Osteoporosis	Bone densitometry (e.g. DEXA) scan	Bisphoshonates
Glaucoma	Measurement of intraocular pressure	Referral for management

steroids may have limited effect of VT burden. Accordingly, it is advised that ICD implantation for VT in CS *not* be deferred for course of steroid therapy [1]. Amiodarone has been used effectively for VT in CS, although controlled studies are lacking. Catheter radiofrequency ablation has been used to reduce the burden of VT in small series of patients [18], but may be less efficacious than when used for VT in other forms of non-ischemic cardiomyopathy [19].

Worsening Systolic Function

Patients presenting with a new decline in LV systolic function, especially without significant dilated remodeling are generally treated aggressively with corticosteroids. As with other forms of cardiomyopathy, once significant dilated remodeling has occurred, the prospects of recovery with therapy (anti-inflammatories in the case of CS) is generally limited. In an uncontrolled retrospective study of CS treated with corticosteroids, including 24 with systolic dysfunction (LVEF <55 %), Chiu et al. reported an improvement in LVEF (40 ± 10–51 ± 12 %, p=0.008) in patients with moderate systolic dysfunction at baseline. However there was no improvement in the subset with severe systolic dysfunction (LVEF <30 %) prior to starting steroids [20]. The time course of recovery of systolic function has not been well described.

Our approach is to consider corticosteroids in patients with severe systolic dysfunction where ventricular dilation is not present and/or where FDG-PET suggests active inflammation. Conversely the absence of inflammation by FDG PET may identify a subset of patients with mild-moderate systolic dysfunction who may not benefit from steroid therapy. Of the different patterns of CS activity on FDG-PET, the presence of a perfusion defect with FDG avidity ("mismatch pattern") and/or right ventricular FDG uptake have been associated with worse prognosis and hence may have the most to benefit from corticosteroid therapy [21]. Sarcoidosis recurrence has been reported in patients who have undergone cardiac transplantation for CS, representing a challenging subset with recurrent disease despite active immunosuppression [22].

Pearls of Wisdom
1. The diagnosis of CS should be considered early in an acute presentation of symptomatic heart disease, as certain therapies (i.e., pacemaker or ICD implantation) can preclude/confound/delay tests used to diagnose CS.
2. Corticosteroid therapy is likely most effective for patients with symptomatic AV block, and may benefit patients with mild systolic dysfunction. Steroid therapy may not benefit patients with symptomatic VT or advanced cardiomyopathy.
3. Prior to initiating corticosteroid therapy for CS, patients should be assessed for side effects and toxicities.

References

1. Birnie DH, Sauer WH, Bogun F, et al. HRS expert consensus statement on the diagnosis and management of arrhythmias associated with cardiac sarcoidosis. Heart Rhythm. 2014;11:1305–23.
2. Diagnostic standard and guidelines for sarcoidosis. Jpn J Sarcoidosis Granulomatous Disord. 2007;27:89–102.
3. Judson MA, Costabel U, Drent M, et al. The WASOG sarcoidosis organ assessment instrument: an update of a previous clinical tool. Sarcoidosis Vasc Diffuse Lung Dis. 2014;31:19–27.
4. Nery PB, Beanlands RS, Nair GM, et al. Atrioventricular block as the initial manifestation of cardiac sarcoidosis in middle-aged adults. J Cardiovasc Electrophysiol. 2014;25:875–81.
5. Koplan BA, Soejima K, Baughman K, Epstein LM, Stevenson WG. Refractory ventricular tachycardia secondary to cardiac sarcoidosis: electrophysiologic characteristics, mapping, and ablation. Heart Rhythm. 2006;3:924–9.
6. Nery PB, Mc Ardle BA, Redpath CJ, Leung E, Lemery R, Dekemp R, Yang J, Keren A, Beanlands RS, Birnie DH. Prevalence of cardiac sarcoidosis in patients presenting with monomorphic ventricular tachycardia. Pacing Clin Electrophysiol. 2014;37:364–74.
7. Hershberger RE, Siegfried JD. Update 2011: clinical and genetic issues in familial dilated cardiomyopathy. J Am Coll Cardiol. 2011;57:1641–9.
8. Lakdawala NK, Givertz MM. Dilated cardiomyopathy with conduction disease and arrhythmia. Circulation. 2010;122:527–34.
9. Saffitz JE. Arrhythmogenic cardiomyopathy: advances in diagnosis and disease pathogenesis. Circulation. 2011;124:e390–2.
10. Lakdawala NK, Funke BH, Baxter S, et al. Genetic testing for dilated cardiomyopathy in clinical practice. J Card Fail. 2012;18:296–303.

11. Lakdawala NK. Using genetic testing to guide therapeutic decisions in cardiomyopathy. Curr Treat Options Cardiovasc Med. 2013;15:387–96.
12. Fox MC, Lakdawala N, Miller AL, Loscalzo J. Clinical problem-solving. A patient with syncope. N Engl J Med. 2013;369:966–72.
13. Viotti R, Vigliano C, Lococo B, Bertocchi G, Petti M, Alvarez MG, Postan M, Armenti A. Long-term cardiac outcomes of treating chronic Chagas disease with benznidazole versus no treatment: a nonrandomized trial. Ann Intern Med. 2006;144:724–34.
14. Lattes R, Lasala MB. Chagas disease in the immunosuppressed patient. Clin Microbiol Infect. 2014;20:300–9.
15. Lee JC, Seiler J, Blankstein R, Padera RF, Baughman KL, Tedrow UB. Images in cardiovascular medicine. Cardiac sarcoidosis presenting as heart block. Circulation. 2009;120:1550–1.
16. Nery PB, Keren A, Healey J, Leug E, Beanlands RS, Birnie DH. Isolated cardiac sarcoidosis: establishing the diagnosis with electroanatomic mapping-guided endomyocardial biopsy. Can J Cardiol. 2013;29:1015.e1–3.
17. Sadek MM, Yung D, Birnie DH, Beanlands RS, Nery PB. Corticosteroid therapy for cardiac sarcoidosis: a systematic review. Can J Cardiol. 2013;29:1034–41.
18. Jefic D, Joel B, Good E, Morady F, Rosman H, Knight B, Bogun F. Role of radiofrequency catheter ablation of ventricular tachycardia in cardiac sarcoidosis: report from a multicenter registry. Heart Rhythm. 2009;6:189–95.
19. Tokuda M, Tedrow UB, Kojodjojo P, Inada K, Koplan BA, Michaud GF, John RM, Epstein LM, Stevenson WG. Catheter ablation of ventricular tachycardia in nonischemic heart disease. Circ Arrhythm Electrophysiol. 2012;5:992–1000.
20. Chiu C-Z, Nakatani S, Zhang G, Tachibana T, Ohmori F, Yamagishi M, Kitakaze M, Tomoike H, Miyatake K. Prevention of left ventricular remodeling by long-term corticosteroid therapy in patients with cardiac sarcoidosis. Am J Cardiol. 2005;95:143–6.
21. Blankstein R, Osborne M, Naya M, et al. Cardiac positron emission tomography enhances prognostic assessments of patients with suspected cardiac sarcoidosis. J Am Coll Cardiol. 2014;63:329–36.
22. Osborne M, Kolli S, Padera RF, Naya M, Lewis E, Dorbala S, Di Carli MF, Blankstein R. Use of multimodality imaging to diagnose cardiac sarcoidosis as well as identify recurrence following heart transplantation. J Nucl Cardiol. 2013;20:310–2.

Chapter 11
Immunosuppressive Management of Cardiac Sarcoidosis

Divya Patel and Nabeel Y. Hamzeh

Abstract Sarcoidosis is a multi-system granulomatous disorder of yet unknown etiology that predominantly involves the lungs in over 90 % of cases but can also involve any organ in the body. Cardiac sarcoidosis is detected clinically in about 5 % of patients with sarcoidosis but on autopsy in as many as 40 % suggesting that the majority of cases may be underdiagnosed. Complications of cardiac sarcoidosis can include ventricular dysfunction, conduction abnormalities, ventricular arrhythmias and sudden cardiac death. These may occur suddenly, without warning in a previously asymptomatic or undiagnosed patient. There are currently no guidelines on how to definitively manage cardiac sarcoidosis. The goal of immunosuppressive (IS) therapy in cardiac sarcoidosis is to reverse any ongoing active granulomatous myocarditis, potentially prevent progression of myocardial granulomatous inflammation to scar tissue, and reduce or prevent the development of serious or life threatening cardiac complications. Management of cardiac sarcoidosis requires the collaborative effort of a sarcoidosis expert, an electrophysiologist, and a general cardiologist.

D. Patel, DO (✉)
Division of Pulmonary and Critical Care Sciences, Department of Medicine,
University of Colorado Hospital, 12401 East 17th Avenue, Aurora, CO, USA
e-mail: divcpatel@gmail.com

N.Y. Hamzeh, MD
Division of Environmental and Occupational Health Sciences, Department of Medicine,
National Jewish Health, 1400 Jackson St., Denver, CO 80206, USA

Division of Pulmonary and Critical Care Sciences, Department of Medicine,
University of Colorado Hospital, 12401 East 17th Avenue, Aurora, CO, USA
e-mail: hamzehn@njhealth.org

© Springer International Publishing Switzerland 2015
A.M. Freeman, H.D. Weinberger (eds.), *Cardiac Sarcoidosis:*
Key Concepts in Pathogenesis, Disease Management, and Interesting Cases,
DOI 10.1007/978-3-319-14624-9_11

Introduction

Sarcoidosis is a multi-system granulomatous disorder of yet unknown etiology [1] which predominantly involves the lungs in over 90 % of cases but can also involve any organ in the body [1, 2]. In the United States, the age-adjusted annual incidence rate in Caucasians is 10.9 per 100,000 and 35.5 per 100,000 in African Americans [1]. Cardiac sarcoidosis is detected clinically in about 5 % of patients with sarcoidosis but on autopsy in as many as 40 % suggesting that it is clinically underdiagnosed [3, 4]. It can be asymptomatic or present as palpitations, dyspnea on exertion out of proportion to pulmonary involvement, syncope or pre-syncopal episodes, or rarely with sudden cardiac death [3, 4]. There are currently no guidelines or statements on how to manage cardiac sarcoidosis [5]. Management of cardiac sarcoidosis requires the collaborative effort of a sarcoidosis expert, an electrophysiologist, and a general cardiologist.

Indication of Immunosuppressive Therapy

The goal of immunosuppressive (IS) therapy in cardiac sarcoidosis is to reverse any ongoing active granulomatous myocarditis and potentially prevent progression of myocardial granulomatous inflammation to scar tissue. The presence of myocardial scar can lead to development of arrhythmias, conduction defects, and/or ventricular dysfunction [6]. Several retrospective studies have shown improvement in conduction defects, ventricular arrhythmias and ventricular dysfunction with IS therapy [7, 8]. However, no randomized prospective studies investigating therapeutics in cardiac sarcoidosis exist. The presence of left ventricular (LV) dysfunction, ventricular arrhythmias, hypermetabolic activity on cardiac 18-fluoro deoxy-glucose positron emission tomography (18-FDG PET), conduction defects, delayed hyper-enhancement on cardiac magnetic resonance imaging, and right ventricular dysfunction in the absence of pulmonary hypertension [5] had a high agreement rate amongst sarcoidosis experts in the United States as an indication for medical treatment.

Impact of IS Therapy on Electrocardiographic Changes

Cardiac sarcoidosis can present with ventricular arrhythmias and/or conduction defects [9]. In a case series of 15 patients diagnosed with cardiac sarcoidosis based on the Japanese Ministry of Health and Welfare (JMHW) criteria, Yodogawa et al. reported improvement of advanced or complete atrioventricular block (AVB) to normal sinus rhythm or first degree AVB in 7 out of 15 patients [10]. The group with improvement in AVB had a statistically significant better baseline left ventricular ejection fraction (LVEF) compared to the group that did not show improvement in their AVB [10]. Yodogawa et al. also retrospectively studied 31 cardiac sarcoidosis patients, diagnosed according to the modified guidelines from the JMHW, with frequent premature ventricular contractions (PVCs >300/day) detected on a 24 h Holter monitor [8]. The cohort was treated with corticosteroids at an equivalent dose of 30 mg/day and tapered over 6 months to a maintenance dose of 10 mg daily [8]. Overall there was no significant difference between the number of PVCs before and after therapy in the entire cohort [8]. However, when grouped based on LV function (LVEF<35 % and LVEF≥35 %); the group with the better LV function showed a statistically significant decrease in the number of PVCs [8]. The group with better LV function also showed a significantly higher prevalence of myocardial gallium-67 uptake, a trend towards an improvement in their LVEF, and an improvement in non-sustained ventricular tachycardia [8]. They also reported that four out of eight patients who had complete AVB had normalization of their complete AVB [8].

Another study examined the impact of corticosteroid therapy in a series of treated and untreated cardiac sarcoidosis patients with normal LVEF and evidence of AVB [11]. Five out of seven patients in the group that received steroid therapy showed resolution of their AVB compared to none in the untreated group (0/13) [11]. During the follow up period, the untreated group showed a marked decline in their LVEF over time and ventricular tachycardia developed in 8 out of 13 in the untreated group compared to only 1 out of 7 in the treated group [11]. Banba et al. showed similar findings in their cohort with improvement or resolution of advanced AVB in 56 % of their cohort with corticosteroid therapy [12].

Impact of IS Therapy on Left Ventricular Function

Chiu et al. retrospectively investigated the effect of corticosteroid therapy on LV function [7]. Forty three cardiac sarcoidosis subjects, prior to initiation of corticosteroid therapy, were divided according to their LVEF into normal (LVEF≥55 %), mild to moderately reduced (LVEF 30–54 %) and severely reduced (LVEF≤30 %) [7]. Patients were treated with prednisolone 30 mg daily or equivalent and tapered to a maintenance dose of 10 mg daily. Patients with normal LVEF and patients with severely reduced LVEF showed no significant changes in their LV function whereas patients with mild to moderately reduced LVEF showed a significant improvement in their LV function [7]. Kato et al. also showed a decline in the LVEF of their untreated group compared to stability of the LVEF in the treated group [11].

Impact of IS Therapy on Survival

The overall survival in cardiac sarcoidosis has been reported to be 98 % after 1 year, 93 % after 3 years, 90 % after 5 years, and 84 % after 10 years but these rates are significantly influenced by other factors [7]. Yazaki et al. investigated the prognostic determinants of survival in cardiac sarcoidosis patients who were treated with corticosteroids [13]. They identified 95 subjects who met the JMHW criteria for the diagnosis of cardiac sarcoidosis [13]. Twenty out of 95 (21.1 %) subjects never received corticosteroids as sarcoidosis was diagnosed on autopsy [13]. Seventy-five out of 95 (78.9 %) were treated with corticosteroids and were classified into a group with normal LV function (EF≥50 %) and a group with reduced LV function (EF<50 %). They were also classified according to the equivalent daily dose of prednisone into a high dose group (≥40 mg/day) and a low dose group (<40 mg/day) [13]. The cohort that did not receive treatment with prednisone and whose diagnosis was discovered on autopsy had a higher incidence of reduced LVEF and a higher incidence of electrocardiographic abnormalities compared to the cohort that received treatment with prednisone [13]. In the group that received prednisone treatment, those who had a LVEF≥50 % had a higher survival rate compared to those who had a LVEF<50 % regardless of the dose of prednisone given (≥40 mg/day versus <40 mg/day) [13]. Multivariable analysis identified New York Heart Association (NYHA) functional class, LV end-diastolic diameter and sustained ventricular tachycardia as independent predictors of mortality [13]. Overall, their findings indicate that LV systolic function and NYHA functional class are predictors of long term prognosis and that high initial doses of prednisone (≥40 mg/day) may not offer any additional benefit compared to lower initial doses [13]. Chiu et al. reported similar findings in their cohort of 43 patients treated with prednisolone [7]. The overall survival was 98 % after 1 year, 93 % after 3 years, 90 % after 5 years, and 84 % after 10 years [7]. However, survival rates differed when analyzed based on LV function [7]. There were no cardiac deaths in the group with preserved LVEF whereas the survival rate in the group with mild to moderately reduced LV function (LVEF 30–54 %) was 100 % after 1, 3, and 5 years and 67 % after 10 years and the survival rate in the group with severely reduced LV function (LVEF<30 %) was worse with 91 % survival after 1 year, 72 % after 3 years, 57 % after 5 years, and 19 % after 10 years [7].

Choice of Agent and Duration of Therapy

To date, all cardiac sarcoidosis therapeutic studies have investigated the use of corticosteroids but one recently published small study investigated the potential role of methotrexate in combination with low dose corticosteroids in cardiac sarcoidosis [14]. This open-label study showed greater stability of LVEF and LV end diastolic diameter in the group that received the combination therapy of low dose methotrexate (6 mg/week) and low dose corticosteroids (5–15 mg/day) compared to corticosteroids alone [14]. No details were provided regarding the tapering schedule of corticosteroids or the difference in the maintenance dose of corticosteroids between the two groups [14]. The patients in this study were treated for a period of 5 years; however, the optimal duration of therapy in cardiac sarcoidosis has yet to be determined.

Anti-TNF-α therapy use in cardiac sarcoidosis has been reported in case reports [15, 16] but their use should be avoided in patients with impaired LV function

(EF ≤ 35 %) as there is an increased risk of adverse events based on studies investigating the role of anti-TNF-α in patients with congestive heart failure from causes other than cardiac sarcoidosis [17].

Expert Consensus

Due to the lack of clear guidelines and literature on the use of immunosuppressive (IS) therapy in cardiac sarcoidosis, we conducted a Delphi study to investigate the approach of physicians in the United States with expertise in sarcoidosis and to investigate if a consensus could be reached on the best approach to manage cardiac sarcoidosis (Table 11.1) [5]. Most experts stated that they would initiate IS therapy when there is evidence of ventricular arrhythmias, hypermetabolic activity on a myocardial FDG-PET scan, conduction defects and/or delayed enhancement on a cardiac MRI [5]. Although over three quarters of the experts would initiate IS therapy for a positive myocardial FDG-PET, less than one quarter would initiate therapy in an asymptomatic patient with only an abnormal FDG-PET and otherwise normal workup [5]. Corticosteroids were the treatment of choice for nearly all the experts and most started prednisone at a dose of 40 mg daily or less and methotrexate was the second most common agent used in the management of cardiac sarcoidosis whereas some reported the use of azathioprine, mycophenolate mofetil and/or anti-tumor necrosis factor-alpha (anti-TNF-α) agents [5]. Table 11.2 outlines pharmacologic agents used in the treatment of sarcoidosis. The majority of the experts use the same dosing regimen regardless of the indication to initiate therapy (arrhythmias vs. cardiomyopathy) but the experts were equally divided on whether to initiate a steroid sparing agent at the same time they initiate corticosteroids [5]. There was little agreement on the duration of therapy in a patient who exhibits an excellent response to IS therapy and several experts mentioned that they utilize the same diagnostic modality that indicated the presence of cardiac sarcoidosis to assess response to therapy [5].

An example case is illustrated in Fig. 11.1 in a woman with neurosarcoidosis who also had cardiac involvement. After IS treatment, her cardiac involvement improved by MRI.

Summary

Myocardial granulomatous inflammation can lead to conduction defects, ventricular arrhythmias and LV dysfunction. The role of IS therapy is to prevent further myocardial involvement with granulomas and the development of scar tissue which can impair LV function and lead to life threatening arrhythmias and conduction abnormalities. Several studies have shown improvement in conduction defects, ventricular arrhythmias and LV function with the use of corticosteroids. The overall prognosis in cardiac

Table 11.1 Management of cardiac sarcoidosis based on a Delphi study of sarcoidosis experts in the United States

Topic	Procedure	N (% endorsing)
Indications for initiation of immunomodulatory therapy	(a) **Hypermetabolic activity on a cardiac FDG-PET scan**	**24 (77.4%)**
	(b) *Delayed enhancement on cardiac MRI*	*19 (61.3%)*
	(c) *Conduction defects*	*21 (67.7%)*
	(d) **LV dysfunction**	**24 (77.4%)**
	(e) *RV dysfunction in the absence of pulmonary hypertension*	*18 (58.1%)*
	(f) **Ventricular arrhythmias**	**24 (77.4%)**
	(g) Atrial arrhythmias	13 (41.9%)
	(h) Other	7 (22.6%)
Immunosuppressive therapies used in treating cardiac sarcoidosis	(a) **Prednisone**	**30 (96.8%)**
	(b) Methotrexate	12 (38.7%)
	(c) Azathioprine	6 (19.4%)
	(d) Mycophenolate mofetil	2 (6.5%)
	(e) Anti-TNF agent	5 (16.1%)
	(f) Other	5 (16.1%)
Dose of prednisone used	(a) 20 mg	4 (12.9%)
	(b) 30–40 mg	14 (45.2%)
	(c) 60 mg	7 (22.6%)
	(d) 0.5 mg/kg/ideal body weight	3 (9.7%)
	(e) 1 mg/kg/ideal body weight	2 (6.5%)
	(f) I don't use prednisone	0 (0%)
	(g) Other	2 (6.5%)
Initiation of steroid sparing agent with corticosteroids	(a) No	11 (42.3%)
	(b) Yes	12 (46.2%)
	(c) Other	4 (15.4%)
Does the initial dosage of steroids differ depending on indication (active arrhythmias versus cardiomyopathy)?	(a) **No, I use the same dosing range no matter what the indication**	**19 (70.4%)**
	(b) Yes, I choose a higher dose for arrhythmias	6 (22.2%)
	(c) Yes, I choose a higher dose for cardiomyopathy	3 (11.1%)
	(d) Other	2 (7.4%)
Duration of immunosuppressive therapy	(a) 1 year	4 (14.8%)
	(b) 2 years	5 (18.5%)
	(c) Indefinitely	7 (25.9%)
	(d) Other	13 (48.1%)
Does the duration of immunosuppressive therapy differ depending on indication (active arrhythmias versus cardiomyopathy)?	(a) *No*	*18 (66.7%)*
	(b) *Yes*	6 (22.2%)
	(c) Other	7 (25.9%)

Bold = Agreement ≥70%, *Italics* = agreement ≥50% but <70%
Abbreviations: *FDG-PET* 18-fluorodeoxyglucose Positron Emission Testing, *cMRI* Cardiac Magnetic Resonance Imaging, *LV* Left Ventricular, *RV* Right Ventricular

Table 11.2 Agents commonly used in the management of sarcoidosis. None of the steroid-sparing agents have been studied in cardiac sarcoidosis

	Recommended dose	Main side-effects	Monitoring needed	Comments
Prednisone	20–30 mg daily or equivalent to be tapered gradually over 6 months	Weight gain, increase blood sugar, hypertension, osteopenia/osteoporosis, infection, neuropsychiatric reactions, infections	Blood sugar, weight, blood pressure, bone density	Rapid-acting but has numerous short and long term side effects
Methotrexate [18]	10–20 mg weekly orally or subcutaneous. Folate supplementation 1–5 mg daily	Gastrointestinal effects, leucopenia, anemia, thrombocytopenia, hepatotoxicity, alopecia, interstitial pneumonitis, infections	Complete blood count, liver function tests, renal function every 1–3 months	No evidence for its use in cardiac sarcoidosis
Azathioprine [19]	50–150 mg/day	Gastrointestinal effects, hepatotoxicity, photosensitivity, infections	Complete blood count and liver function tests every 1–3 months. Check thiopurine S-methyltransferase function	No evidence for its use in cardiac sarcoidosis
Leflunomide [20]	10–20 mg/day	Gastrointestinal effects, diarrhea, hepatotoxicity, neutropenia, neuropathy, hypertension, infections	Complete blood count and renal function tests every 1–3 months	No evidence for its use in cardiac sarcoidosis
Mycophenolate mofetil [21]	500–3,000 mg/day	Neutropenia, gastrointestinal effects, diarrhea, headaches, infections	Complete blood count and liver function tests every 1–3 months. Check thiopurine S-methyltransferase function	No evidence for its use in cardiac sarcoidosis
TNF-α antagonist [22]	Infliximab 3–5 mg per kg intravenously at week 0, 2, 6, then every 4–8 weeks	Allergic and infusion reactions, risk of serious infections including tuberculosis and fungal	Assessment for latent tuberculosis infection	No evidence for its use in cardiac sarcoidosis. Contraindicated in patients with low ejection fraction

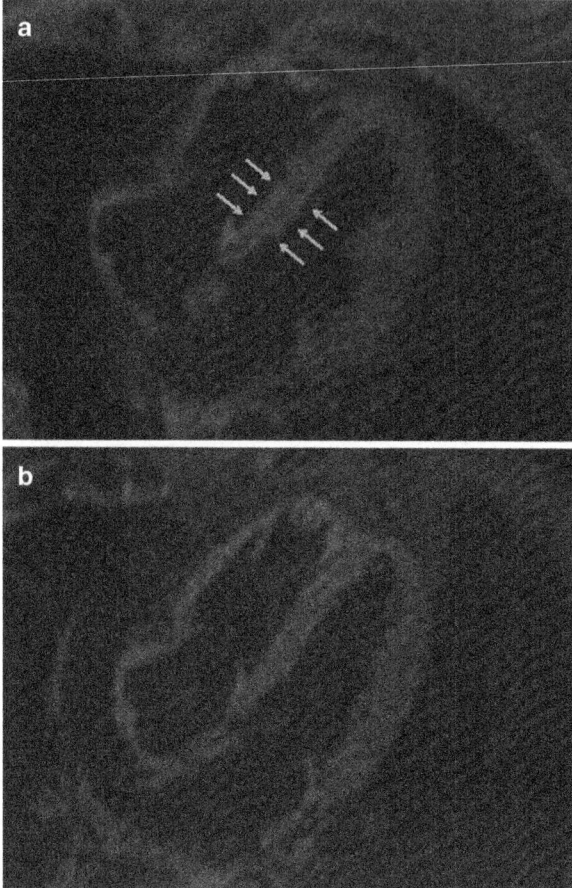

Fig. 11.1 (**a**) Before immunosuppressive therapy. (**b**) After immunosuppressive therapy. Fifty-four year old female patient with neurosarcoidosis underwent cardiac MRI with and without gadolinium for evaluation of suspected cardiac sarcoidosis. Following standard localizing images, T2 weighted dark blood images were obtained at 5 mm slice thickness from the pulmonary artery to the inferior aspect of the heart. Perpendicular, horizontal and short axis images were obtained using a single breath-hold trueFISP gated cine technique. T2 weighted dark blood images and STIR imaging were performed in short and horizontal long axis. In the interventricular septum, focal punctuate areas of enhancement within the epicardial portion of the inferoseptal wall were seen before immunosuppressive therapy (**a**). She received corticosteroids for a year and had a repeat cardiac MRI 1 year later showed complete resolution of the focal punctuate areas of enhancement in the interventricular septum and no evidence of delayed hyperenhancement (**b**)

sarcoidosis is impacted by LV function and NYHA functional class of the patient. The use of high dose corticosteroids (>40 mg daily) did not offer additional benefit compared to a dose of 40 mg daily or less and the role of steroid sparing agents in sarcoidosis has yet to be formerly studied although they are used in the management of cardiac sarcoidosis. The optimal duration of therapy is unknown but should be guided by the extent of cardiac involvement and the nature of response to therapy.

Pearls of Wisdom
1. Cardiac sarcoidosis is under diagnosed ante-mortem, and a high index of suspicion to look for evidence of myocardial involvement should be maintained in patients with sarcoidosis.
2. Goals of therapy are to reduce and/or prevent permanent myocardial damage and the significant and life threatening complications of cardiomyopathy and heart failure, conduction abnormalities including complete heart block, and ventricular arrhythmias and sudden cardiac death.
3. Prednisone is the only agent that has been studied in the treatment of cardiac sarcoidosis, but other immunosuppressive therapies are often used, but have not yet been formally studied.

References

1. Statement on sarcoidosis. Am J Respir Crit Care Med. 1999;160(2):736–55.
2. Baughman RP, Teirstein AS, Judson MA, Rossman MD, Yeager H, Brenitz EA, et al. Clinical characteristics of patients in a case control study of sarcoidosis. Am J Respir Crit Care Med. 2001;164:1885–9.
3. Silverman KJ, Hutchins GM, Bulkley BH. Cardiac sarcoid: a clinicopathologic study of 84 unselected patients with systemic sarcoidosis. Circulation. 1978;58(6):1204–11.
4. Mehta D, Lubitz SA, Frankel Z, Wisnivesky JP, Einstein AJ, Goldman M, et al. Cardiac involvement in patients with sarcoidosis: diagnostic and prognostic value of outpatient testing. Chest. 2008;133(6):1426–35.
5. Hamzeh NY, Wamboldt FS, Weinberger HD. Management of cardiac sarcoidosis in the United States: a Delphi study. Chest. 2012;141(1):154–62.
6. Ayyala US, Nair AP, Padilla ML. Cardiac sarcoidosis. Clin Chest Med. 2008;29(3):493–508, ix.
7. Chiu C-Z, Nakatani S, Zhang G, Tachibana T, Ohmori F, Yamagishi M, et al. Prevention of left ventricular remodeling by long-term corticosteroid therapy in patients with cardiac sarcoidosis. Am J Cardiol. 2005;95(1):143–6.
8. Yodogawa K, Seino Y, Ohara T, Takayama H, Katoh T, Mizuno K. Effect of corticosteroid therapy on ventricular arrhythmias in patients with cardiac sarcoidosis. Ann Noninvasive Electrocardiol. 2011;16(2):140–7.
9. Doughan AR, Williams BR. Cardiac sarcoidosis. Heart (British Cardiac Society). 2006;92(2):282–8.
10. Yodogawa K, Seino Y, Shiomura R, Takahashi K, Tsuboi I, Uetake S, et al. Recovery of atrioventricular block following steroid therapy in patients with cardiac sarcoidosis. J Cardiol. 2013;62(5):320–5.
11. Kato Y, Morimoto S, Uemura A, Hiramitsu S, Ito T, Hishida H. Efficacy of corticosteroids in sarcoidosis presenting with atrioventricular block. Sarcoidosis Vasc Diffuse Lung Dis. 2003;20(2):133–7.
12. Banba K, Kusano KF, Nakamura K, Morita H, Ogawa A, Ohtsuka F, et al. Relationship between arrhythmogenesis and disease activity in cardiac sarcoidosis. Heart Rhythm. 2007;4(10):1292–9.
13. Yazaki Y, Isobe M, Hiroe M, Morimoto S, Hiramitsu S, Nakano T, et al. Prognostic determinants of long-term survival in Japanese patients with cardiac sarcoidosis treated with prednisone. Am J Cardiol. 2001;88(9):1006–10.
14. Nagai S, Yokomatsu T, Tanizawa K, Ikezoe K, Handa T, Ito Y, et al. Treatment with methotrexate and low-dose corticosteroids in sarcoidosis patients with cardiac lesions. Intern Med. 2014;53(5):427–33.

15. Barnabe C, McMeekin J, Howarth A, Martin L. Successful treatment of cardiac sarcoidosis with infliximab. J Rheumatol. 2008;35(8):1686–7.
16. Uthman I, Touma Z, Khoury M. Cardiac sarcoidosis responding to monotherapy with infliximab. Clin Rheumatol. 2007;26(11):2001–3.
17. Chung ES, Packer M, Lo KH, Fasanmade AA, Willerson JT, Investigators ftA. Randomized, double-blind, placebo-controlled, pilot trial of infliximab, a chimeric monoclonal antibody to tumor necrosis factor-α, in patients with moderate-to-severe heart failure: results of the Anti-TNF Therapy Against Congestive Heart failure (ATTACH) trial. Circulation. 2003;107(25): 3133–40.
18. Lower EE, Baughman RP. Prolonged use of methotrexate for sarcoidosis. Arch Intern Med. 1995;155:846–51.
19. Vorselaars AD, Wuyts WA, Vorselaars VM, et al. Methotrexate vs azathioprine in second-line therapy of sarcoidosis. Chest. 2013;144:805–12.
20. Baughman RP, Lower EE. Leflunomide for chronic sarcoidosis. Sarcoidosis Vasc Diffuse Lung Dis. 2004;21:43–8.
21. Androdias G, Maillet D, Marignier R, et al. Mycophenolate mofetil may be effective in CNS sarcoidosis but not in sarcoid myopathy. Neurology. 2011;76:1168–72.
22. Baughman RP, Lower EE. Infliximab for refractory sarcoidosis. Sarcoidosis Vasc Diffuse Lung Dis. 2001;18:70–4.

Chapter 12
Management of Sudden Death Risk Related to Cardiac Sarcoidosis

Matthew M. Zipse and William H. Sauer

Abstract The most feared complication of cardiac sarcoidosis (CS) is sudden cardiac death (SCD) resulting from ventricular arrhythmias. SCD accounts for 30–65 % of deaths in sarcoidosis and may be its first manifestation. Once cardiac involvement is suspected or identified, efforts should be made to further stratify a patient's risk of sudden cardiac death by some combination of ECG, electrophysiologic testing, echocardiogram, and advanced imaging. In addition to a LVEF ≤35 %, high risk features such as need for permanent pacing, mild to moderately reduced LV systolic function (LVEF 36–49 %) or reduced RV systolic function (RVEF <40 %), or inducible VT by EP study are indications for ICD implantation. Patients should be followed closely over time as those without initial indications of cardiac involvement or need for ICD may develop such in the future. This chapter will focus on the role of the ICD in CS in addition to risk stratification in those at risk for SCD with CS.

Introduction

The most feared complication of cardiac sarcoidosis (CS) is sudden cardiac death (SCD) resulting from ventricular arrhythmias. SCD accounts for 30–65 % of deaths in sarcoidosis [1–3]. Unfortunately, not only are ventricular arrhythmias and sudden death common in CS, but many times they present as the first clinical manifestation of CS [2, 4]. For this reason, a high index of suspicion and low threshold to screen for myocardial involvement are paramount.

After the diagnosis of CS is made, an implantable cardiac defibrillator (ICD) may be indicated as part of the management of SCD risk (Table 12.1 and Fig. 12.1) [5]. This chapter will focus on the role of the ICD in CS.

M.M. Zipse, MD • W.H. Sauer, MD (✉)
Section of Cardiac Electrophysiology, Division of Cardiology, University of Colorado Hospital, 12401 East 17th Avenue, B136, Aurora, CO 80045, USA
e-mail: Matthew.Zipse@ucdenver.edu; william.sauer@ucdenver.edu

© Springer International Publishing Switzerland 2015
A.M. Freeman, H.D. Weinberger (eds.), *Cardiac Sarcoidosis:*
Key Concepts in Pathogenesis, Disease Management, and Interesting Cases,
DOI 10.1007/978-3-319-14624-9_12

Table 12.1 Expert consensus recommendations for implantation cardioverter defibrillators in patients with CS [5]

Class I Recommendation
ICD implantation is recommended in patients with CS and one or more of the following:
1. Spontaneous sustained ventricular arrhythmias, including prior cardiac arrest.
2. The LVEF is ≤35 %, despite optimal medical therapy and a period of immunosuppression (if there is active inflammation).
Class IIa Recommendation
ICD implantation can be useful in patients with CS, independent of ventricular function and one or more of the following:
1. An indication for permanent pacemaker implantation.
2. Unexplained syncope or near-syncope, felt to be arrhythmic in etiology.
3. Inducible sustained ventricular arrhythmias (>30 s of monomorphic VT or polymorphic VT) or clinically relevant ventricular fibrillation[a].
Class IIb Recommendation
ICD implantation may be considered in patients with LVEF 36–49 % and/or an RV ejection fraction <40 %, despite optimal medical therapy and a period of immunosuppression (if there is active inflammation).
Class III Recommendations
ICD implantation is not recommended in patients with no history of syncope, normal LVEF/RVEF, no LGE on CMR, a negative EP Study and no indication for permanent pacing. However, these patients should be closely followed for deterioration in ventricular function.
ICD implantation is not recommended in patients with one or more of the following:
1. Incessant ventricular arrhythmias.
2. Severe NYHA class IV heart failure.

[a]Ventricular fibrillation with triple premature beats of less than 220 ms is considered a nonspecific response

Risk Stratification

While some electrophysiologists will chose to implant a primary prevention ICD in all patients with cardiac sarcoidosis, most agree that further risk stratification is needed to discern who may benefit from the ICD, as some CS patients appear to follow a fairly benign clinical course. In fact, by the most recent expert consensus guidelines, the ICD is contraindicated (Class III recommendation) in patients with no history of syncope, normal ventricular function, no evidence of delayed contrast enhancement on cardiac magnetic resonance imaging (CMRI), a negative electrophysiology (EP) study, and with no indication for pacing [5]. Ultimately, risk stratification may be guided by a combination of CMRI and 18-FDG myocardial positron emission tomography (PET) findings, electrophysiologic testing with programmed electrical stimulation, or by other high risk clinical features such as atrioventricular block, systolic dysfunction, or a history of syncope. Current guidelines recognize the paucity of randomized, prospective data, and cite the limitations of retrospectively analyzed series; ultimately, further research is needed to better advise practice.

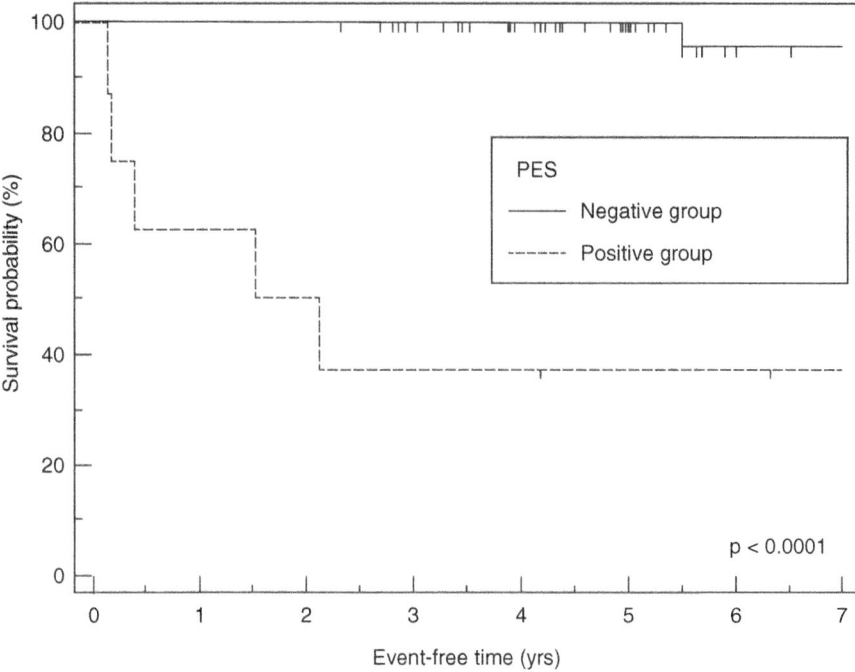

Fig. 12.1 Kaplan-Meier estimation of event free survival as stratified by programmed electrical stimulation by EP study. *Vertical markers* indicate the time when follow-up was terminated in each patient [20]. *PES* programmed electrical stimulation

Sudden Death Risk Stratification by LV and RV Systolic Function

Due to both the element of active granulomatous inflammation, and the heterogenous involvement of the left ventricle (LV) and/or right ventricle (RV), CS may behave differently than other cardiomyopathies when it comes to risk of ventricular arrhythmias and SCD. Accordingly, a different set of rules may govern SCD risk and ICD indications than the standard LVEF <35 % that is often used for non-sarcoidosis cardiomyopathies. While CS patients with EF <35 % should receive a primary prevention ICD in accordance with accepted device guidelines [6], many CS patients with EF >35 % may also be candidates for primary prevention ICD implantation.

While a lower LVEF is associated with appropriate ICD therapy in several retrospective studies, many patients with only mildly impaired LV function also had substantial risk of ventricular arrhythmias and resultant appropriate ICD shocks and anti-tachycardia pacing [7–9]. In fact, in the study by Kron et al. most primary and secondary prevention patients who received appropriate ICD therapies had an LVEF >35 %, suggesting that CS patients with mild or moderately reduced LVEF may still be at substantial risk for ventricular arrhythmias [7]. Furthermore, in the study by Betensky et al. 7 of the 17 patients (41 %) with appropriate ICD therapy had LVEF >35 % [9]. While these studies noted that a number of patients with mild and moderately reduced LVEF received appropriate ICD therapies for VT/VF, Schuller et al. reported that in their primary prevention cohort, no patient with normal left and right ventricular systolic function (LVEF >50 % and RVEF >40 %) required ICD therapies over the follow up period [8]. It is from these data that a Class IIa recommendation for consideration of ICD implantation in patients with LVEF 36–49 % and/or RV ejection fraction <40 %, after optimal medical therapy and initiation of immunosuppression if indicated was based.

Sudden Death Risk Stratification with Cardiac Imaging

As discussed in Chaps. 5, 6, and 7, CMRI and 18-FDG myocardial PET appear to be the imaging modalities with the highest sensitivity and specificity in the detection of CS [10–14]. CMRI, in particular, has emerged as the test of choice at many centers in the evaluation of CS, owing in part to a lower false positive rate. CMRI uses T-2 weighted signal and early gadolinium images to detect acute inflammation and late gadolinium enhancement (LGE, also known as delayed contrast enhancement) to assess for fibrosis or scar. Preliminary data also suggest that surveillance with CMRI can assess the efficacy of steroid therapy [15, 16].

Importantly, CMRI has a role in risk stratification and prognosis. In a recent study of 155 consecutive patients with systemic sarcoidosis who underwent CMR for workup of suspected CS, LGE was present in 39 patients (25.5 %), and its presence was associated with a Cox hazard ratio of 31.6 for death, aborted sudden cardiac death, or appropriate ICD discharge [17] over a median 2.6 year follow-up period. Of the twelve patients with sudden cardiac death or appropriate ICD discharge in this study, all had LGE present on CMRI. Sarcoidosis patients without LGE, even those with LV dilatation and severely impaired LVEF, did not experience SCD, suggesting CMRI may provide prognostic data beyond that conferred by ejection fraction alone.

While CMRI may have a higher specificity, ^{18}F-fluoro-2-deoxyglucose positron emission tomography (^{18}F-FDG PET) appears to detect active inflammation in CS with a slightly higher sensitivity [18, 19]. However, as the uptake of ^{18}F-FDG is seen in other inflammatory myocardial diseases, PET is non-specific for CS and must be interpreted in the appropriate clinical context. Like CMRI, PET carries prognostic value – in a study of 118 patients with suspected CS, 60 % had abnormal cardiac PET findings. Over a median follow-up of 1.5 years, abnormal PET findings were associated with a hazard ratio of 3.9 for death or VT, and an abnormal PET remained a significant predictor of death or VT even after multivariate analysis to adjust for ejection fraction and other clinical variables [13], indicating PET offers prognostic value beyond EF alone.

Sudden Death Risk Stratification with Electrophysiologic Testing

Electrophysiologic study can add useful diagnostic information, particularly if CMRI or PET are inconclusive or unable to be obtained. Electroanatomical mapping, or "voltage-mapping," of the right ventricle can help identify areas of scar, which can aid in the diagnosis of CS in the right clinical context. There have also been limited studies investigating the role for programmed electrical stimulation (PES) for the inducibility of sustained monomorphic ventricular tachycardia as a means of risk stratification of sudden cardiac death in patients with CS. One such study of 76 patients with CS undergoing PES showed that 6 of 8 patients (75 %) with inducible VT went on to have ventricular arrhythmias and ICD therapies, compared to 1 patient with sudden cardiac death amongst the 68 patients (1.5 %) who had been non-inducible by PES [20]. In another study of 32 patients with CS, 4 of 6 patients (67 %) with inducible VT went on to have appropriate ICD therapies while 2 of 20 patients (10 %) who were non-inducible went on to have ventricular arrhythmias or sudden cardiac death [21]. While these studies suggest a potential role for electrophysiologic testing in risk stratification, these data ultimately need to be replicated in larger cohorts. Furthermore, these studies are limited by mean follow-up periods of 5 years and 2.6 years, respectively; and, in light of CS as a progressive disease, the long-term prognostic value of a single negative EP study is unclear.

Indications for Implantable Cardiac Defibrillator Therapy

The ACC/AHA/HRS 2008 guidelines give a Class IIA recommendation (level of evidence C) for ICD therapy in sarcoidosis patients with evidence of myocardial involvement, regardless of symptoms or presentation [22]. As discussed earlier in this chapter, HRS released an expert consensus statement in 2014 further refining the specific recommendations for ICD therapy as they pertain to patients with CS (Table 12.1) [5]. Class I indications stand for secondary prevention devices and for those with severe LV dysfunction despite a period of optimal medical therapy as per recommendations for patients with other cardiomyopathies [6]. These guidelines also give Class II recommendations for ICD implantation in CS if there are other features considered to be higher risk (e.g., need for permanent pacing, mild to moderately reduced LV (i.e., LVEF 36–49 %) or RV (i.e., RVEF <40 %) systolic function, or inducible VT by EP study.

These recommendations come at a time when practice patterns are heterogenous [23], with some centers tending to implant ICDs in CS patients only with Class I indications (prior ventricular arrhythmias or LVEF ≤ 35 %), while other centers are offering ICDs to all CS patients (in accordance with the IIA recommendation from the 2008 guidelines). And, while the type of patient for which the primary prevention ICD will benefit does remain controversial in CS, what is becoming evident from a number of observational studies is that among those CS patients who do receive ICDs, both appropriate and inappropriate ICD therapies are common.

Studies of ICD Therapies in CS

Four observational studies were published in 2012–2013 that reported on ICD therapies in patients with CS. Betensky et al. reviewed 45 patients (64 % primary prevention, 2.6 year mean follow-up period), and found a high annualized appropriate therapy (shock and/or anti-tachycardia pacing) rate of 14.5 % [9]. Predictors of appropriate therapies included lower LVEF and complete heart block, signifying more advanced disease. Schuller et al. reported on 112 patients (74 % primary prevention, 2.8 year mean follow-up period) and found a similarly high annualized therapy rate of 13.2 % [8]. Interestingly, in this cohort, no primary prevention patient with normal left and right ventricular systolic function (LVEF > 50 % and RVEF > 40 %) required an ICD therapy, though there were many patients with only mild systolic dysfunction who received shocks and ATP [8]. Mohsen et al. found an annualized therapy rate of 9.6 % in their mixed cohort of primary and secondary prevention CS patients. Interestingly, the rate of inappropriate ICD therapies was quite high (30 % over 3.75 year mean follow-up duration) [24]. Kron et al. published a multicenter retrospective review of 235 patients (99 of which were included in the aforementioned studies), and found male gender, syncope, lower LVEF, and high proportion of ventricular pacing each to be independent risk factors for appropriate therapies (with an annualized incidence of 8.6 % in this study) [7]. Altogether, the rates of appropriate therapies in these three studies are notably higher than that observed in large primary prevention ICD trials such as SCD-HeFT (Sudden Cardiac Death in Heart Failure Trial), where the incidence was approximately 5 % per year [25].

Special Considerations for Post-implant ICD Management in Patients with Cardiac Sarcoidosis

Experience taking care of CS patients with ICDs has brought some special considerations to light. First, as highlighted by the four aforementioned studies, the burden of ventricular arrhythmias is high, as is the annualized rate of appropriate therapies. Chapter 9 discussed the many mechanisms of ventricular arrhythmias in these patients, as well as the high prevalence of electrical storm (Fig. 12.2) [8]. Also noteworthy is the high rate of inappropriate therapies (30 % of patients in the study by Moshen et al. for example) [24], perhaps owing in part to the high burden of atrial arrhythmias in CS (Chap. 12).

Patients with CS and ICDs also have a high incidence of late reduction of sensed R-waves. A nested case-control study on a cohort of 46 patients with CS and ICDs compared to 117 controls with other cardiomyopathies showed that patients with CS have a high incidence of significant (greater than 50 %) reduction in measured electrograms (HR 9.10, 95 % CI 2.50–33.06, Fig. 12.3) [26]. It is possible that local

Fig. 12.2 Pie chart for appropriate therapy [8]

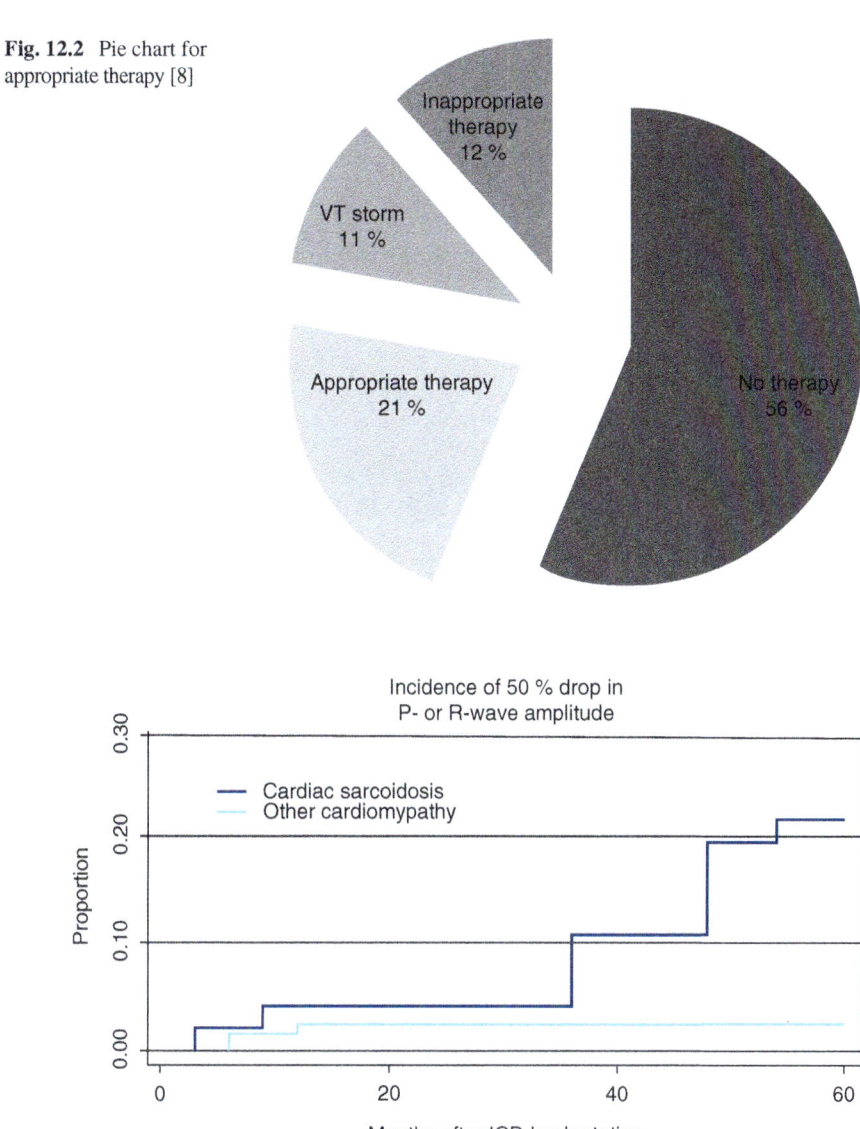

Fig. 12.3 The incidence of 50 % reduction in P or R wave sensing amplitude in CS patients with ICDs. After 5 years of follow-up, 22 % of patients with CS and an ICD had a 50 % or more reduction in measured sensed electrograms on device interrogation, compared to 3 % of patients with ICDs for other forms of cardiomyopathy ($P<0.001$) [26]

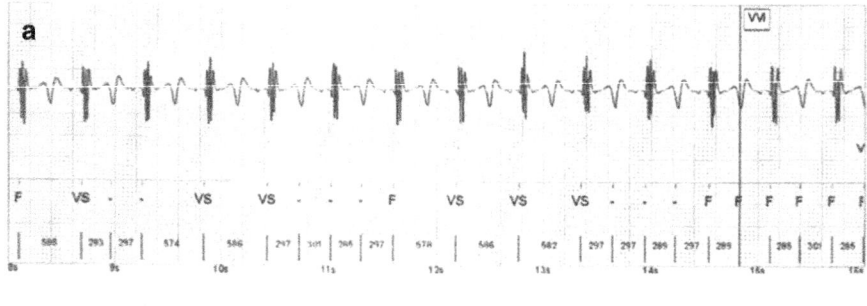

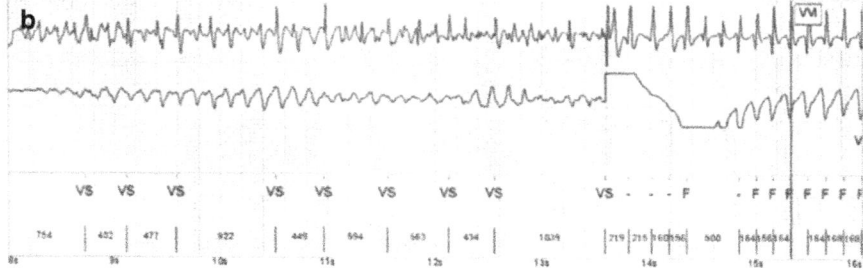

Fig. 12.4 Reductions in sensed R-waves from ICDs in patients with CS can lead to VF under-sensing and failure to deliver appropriate shocks (**a**) as well as T-wave over-sensing (**b**) and the potential delivery of inappropriate shocks

characteristics at the lead tip to tissue interface over time (e.g., inflammation from local granuloma formation) could lead to these reductions in sensing, though the mechanism is unknown. Nonetheless, reductions in sensing can lead to significant clinical consequences, such as under-sensing of VF and failure to deliver appropriate therapies, and over-sensing of T-waves with the delivery of inappropriate therapies (Fig. 12.4). Measured R-waves by the ICD should be followed over time and should prompt DFT testing if reductions in R-waves are significant, and may require lead revision if DFT testing fails.

Lastly, because patients with CS have a high incidence of atrioventricular block, many patients may either meet an indication for a biventricular ICD at the time of initial implant, or may meet an indication for upgrade at the time of generator change if the burden of RV pacing is considerable, as supported by data from the BLOCK HF clinical trial [27].

Conclusion

Upon diagnosis of CS, efforts should be made to further stratify a patient's risk of sudden cardiac death by some combination of ECG, electrophysiologic testing, echocardiogram, and advanced imaging. Many patients with CS will have a Class I, Class IIa, or Class IIb indication for a primary prevention ICD by recent guidelines, and those with a history of VT/VF or aborted sudden cardiac death clearly require an ICD.

Special considerations should be made in the follow-up of CS patients with ICDs, given their high risk of receiving both appropriate and inappropriate shocks. Medications and/or catheter ablation may be required for arrhythmia control. Device parameters, specifically sensed electrograms, should be followed over time and should prompt DFT testing if reductions in R-waves are significant and lead revision if necessary. Ultimately, early referral of newly-diagnosed patients with CS to an electrophysiologist is necessary to aid in initial risk assessment, and ongoing follow-up in device clinic is critical for the continued care of CS patients with ICDs.

Pearls of Wisdom
1. Patients with cardiac sarcoidosis with mild to moderately reduced left ventricular systolic function (LVEF 36–49 %) or reduced right ventricular systolic function (RVEF <40 %) have an increased risk of ventricular arrhythmias and sudden cardiac death and are appropriate to consider for ICD therapy.
2. Patients with cardiac sarcoidosis without initial indications for an ICD should be monitored and followed closely over time for changes and the development of indications for an ICD.
3. Involvement of an electrophysiologist is important in the evaluation, monitoring and management of patients with cardiac sarcoidosis.
4. Advanced imaging including cardiac MRI and 18FDG myocardial PET as well as electrophysiologic studies are important components in the evaluation of risk for serious or life threatening conduction abnormalities, ventricular arrhythmias and sudden cardiac death.

References

1. Roberts WC, McAllister HA, Ferrans VJ. Sarcoidosis of the heart. A clinicopathologic study of 35 necropsy patients (group 1) and review of 78 previously described necropsy patients (group 11). Am J Med. 1977;63:86–108.
2. Matsui Y, Iwai K, Tachibana T, Fruie T, Shigematsu N, Izumi T, et al. Clinicopathological study of fatal myocardial sarcoidosis. Ann N Y Acad Sci. 1976;278:455–69.
3. Fleming HA, Bailey SM. Sarcoid heart disease. J R Coll Physicians Lond. 1981;15:245.
4. Lubitz SA, Goldbarg SH, Mehta D. Sudden cardiac death in infiltrative cardiomyopathies: sarcoidosis, scleroderma, amyloidosis, hemachromatosis. Prog Cardiovasc Dis. 2008;51: 58–73.
5. Birnie DH, Sauer W, Bogun F, Cooper J, Culver DA, Duvernoy C, et al. Heart rhythm society expert consensus statement on the diagnosis and management of arrhythmias associated with cardiac sarcoidosis. HRTHM. 2014;11(7):1304–23. Elsevier.
6. Epstein AE, DiMarco JP, Ellenbogen KA, Estes NAM, Freedman RA, Gettes LS, et al. ACCF/AHA/HRS focused update incorporated into the ACCF/AHA/HRS 2008 guidelines for device-based therapy of cardiac rhythm abnormalities: a report of the American College of Cardiology

Foundation/American Heart Association Task Force on Practice Guidelines and the Heart Rhythm Society. Circulation. 2012;2013:e283–352.
7. Kron J, Sauer W, Schuller J, Bogun F, Crawford T, Sarsam S, et al. Efficacy and safety of implantable cardiac defibrillators for treatment of ventricular arrhythmias in patients with cardiac sarcoidosis. Europace. 2013;15:347–54.
8. Schuller JL, Zipse M, Crawford T, Bogun F, Beshai J, Patel AR, et al. Implantable cardioverter defibrillator therapy in patients with cardiac sarcoidosis. J Cardiovasc Electrophysiol. 2012; 23:925–9.
9. Betensky BP, Tschabrunn CM, Zado ES, Goldberg LR, Marchlinski FE, Garcia FC, et al. Long-term follow-up of patients with cardiac sarcoidosis and implantable cardioverter-defibrillators. Heart Rhythm. 2012;9:884–91. Elsevier Inc.
10. Kim JS, Judson MA, Donnino R, Gold M, Cooper LT, Prystowsky EN, et al. Cardiac sarcoidosis. Am Heart J. 2009;157:9–21.
11. Soejima K, Yada H. The work-up and management of patients with apparent or subclinical cardiac sarcoidosis: with emphasis on the associated heart rhythm abnormalities. J Cardiovasc Electrophysiol. 2009;20:578–83. Wiley Online Library.
12. Youssef G, Beanlands RSB, Birnie DH, Nery PB. Cardiac sarcoidosis: applications of imaging in diagnosis and directing treatment. Heart. 2011;97:2078–87.
13. Blankstein R, Osborne M, Naya M, Waller A, Kim CK, Murthy VL, et al. Cardiac positron emission tomography enhances prognostic assessments of patients with suspected cardiac sarcoidosis. J Am Coll Cardiol. 2014;63:329–36.
14. Ohira H, Tsujino I, Ishimaru S, Oyama N, Takei T, Tsukamoto E, et al. Myocardial imaging with 18F-fluoro-2-deoxyglucose positron emission tomography and magnetic resonance imaging in sarcoidosis. Eur J Nucl Med Mol Imaging. 2008;35:933–41. Springer.
15. Vignaux O, Dhote R, Duboc D, Blanche P, Dusser D, Weber S, et al. Clinical significance of myocardial magnetic resonance abnormalities in patients with sarcoidosis: a 1-year follow-up study. Chest. 2002;122:1895–901.
16. Sekiguchi M, Yazaki Y, Isobe M, Hiroe M. Cardiac sarcoidosis: diagnostic, prognostic, and therapeutic considerations. Cardiovasc Drugs Ther. 1996;10:495–510.
17. Greulich S, Deluigi CC, Gloekler S, Wahl A, Zürn C, Kramer U, et al. CMR imaging predicts death and other adverse events in suspected cardiac sarcoidosis. JACC Cardiovasc Imaging. 2013;6:501–11. Elsevier Inc.
18. Ishimaru S, Tsujino I, Sakaue S, Oyama N, Takei T, Tsukamoto E, et al. Combination of 18F-fluoro-2-deoxyglucose positron emission tomography and magnetic resonance imaging in assessing cardiac sarcoidosis. Sarcoidosis Vasc Diffuse Lung Dis. 2005;22:234–5.
19. Youssef G, Leung E, Mylonas I, Nery P, Williams K, Wisenberg G, et al. The use of 18F-FDG PET in the diagnosis of cardiac sarcoidosis: a systematic review and metaanalysis including the Ontario experience. J Nucl Med. 2012;53:241–8.
20. Mehta D, Mori N, Goldbarg SH, Lubitz S, Wisnivesky JP, Teirstein A. Primary prevention of sudden cardiac death in silent cardiac sarcoidosis: role of programmed ventricular stimulation. Circ Arrhythm Electrophysiol. 2011;4:43–8.
21. Aizer A, Stern EH, Gomes JA, Teirstein AS, Eckart RE, Mehta D. Usefulness of programmed ventricular stimulation in predicting future arrhythmic events in patients with cardiac sarcoidosis. Am J Cardiol. 2005;96:276–82.
22. Writing Committee Members, Epstein AE, DiMarco JP, Ellenbogen KA, Estes NAM, Freedman RA, et al. ACC/AHA/HRS 2008 guidelines for device-based therapy of cardiac rhythm abnormalities: executive summary: a report of the American College of Cardiology/American Heart Association Task Force on Practice Guidelines (Writing Committee to Revise the ACC/AHA/NASPE 2002 Guideline Update for Implantation of Cardiac Pacemakers and Antiarrhythmia Devices): developed in collaboration with the American Association for Thoracic Surgery and Society of Thoracic Surgeons. Circulation. 2008; 117:2820–40.

23. Hamzeh NY, Wamboldt FS, Weinberger HD. Management of cardiac sarcoidosis in the United States: a Delphi study. Chest. 2012;141(1):154–62.
24. Mohsen A, Jimenez A, Hood RE, Dickfeld T, Saliaris A, Shorofsky S, et al. Cardiac sarcoidosis: electrophysiological outcomes on long-term follow-up and the role of the implantable cardioverter-defibrillator. J Cardiovasc Electrophysiol. 2014;25(2):171–6.
25. Bardy GH, Lee KL, Mark DB, Poole JE, Packer DL, Boineau R, et al. Amiodarone or an implantable cardioverter–defibrillator for congestive heart failure. N Engl J Med. 2005; 352:225–37.
26. Zipse MM, Varosy PD, Schuller JL, Steckman DA, Katz DF, Gonzalez JE, et al. Patients with cardiac sarcoidosis and ICDs have a high incidence of late reduction of measured electrograms. Heart Rhythm. 2013;10(5S):S301.
27. Curtis AB, Worley SJ, Adamson PB, Chung ES, Niazi I, Sherfesee L, et al. Biventricular pacing for atrioventricular block and systolic dysfunction. N Engl J Med. 2013;368:1585–93.

Chapter 13
Sarcoidosis-Associated Pulmonary Hypertension

Brett Fenster

Abstract In addition to the myriad of potential clinical presentations of cardiac sarcoidosis, one of the least recognized but perhaps one of the more clinically important ones is sarcoidosis-associated pulmonary hypertension (SAPH), considered part of the World Health Organization class V (multifactorial). The prevalence of sarcoidosis-associated pulmonary hypertension (SAPH) is 5–15 %, and is felt to be multifactorial. It is usually seen in patients with more radiographically severe pulmonary sarcoidosis. The potential consequences of untreated pulmonary hypertension could include the development of right heart failure (cor pulmonale), progressive and refractor shortness of breath, hypoxemia, and even death. Screening and surveillance should be performed for this entity with prompt recognition and treatment to prevent the more serious manifestations. Although there is a growing body of evidence to suggest possible benefit of PAH-specific therapies in SAPH, there are no currently FDA approved medications for SAPH.

Introduction

The recent development of numerous pharmacologic agents for the treatment of pulmonary arterial hypertension (PAH) has spawned a renewed interest in all forms of pulmonary hypertension (PH), including sarcoidosis-associated pulmonary hypertension (SAPH). Although previously thought to be an uncommon complication of chronic pulmonary sarcoidosis, SAPH is now appreciated as an important disease state unto itself that significantly impacts morbidity and mortality. Equally relevant is the recognition that SAPH can be present without or without interstitial lung disease, highlighting the multifactorial etiology of what is likely a diverse set of sarcoidosis-related diseases with the common manifestation of elevated

---

B. Fenster, MD, FACC, FACP, FASE
Division of Cardiology, Department of Medicine, National Jewish Health,
1400 Jackson St., Denver, CO 80206, USA
e-mail: fensterb@njhealth.org

pulmonary pressure. This chapter will discuss the current understanding of SAPH including its prevalence, pathophysiology, treatment, and prognosis.

Epidemiology

Although pulmonary involvement is present in greater than 90 % of sarcoidosis patients, the prevalence of SAPH appears to be closer to 5–15 % [1–3]. While the pathologic and clinical relevance of exercise-associated PH remains controversial, exercise-induced pathologic elevations in pulmonary pressures were present in 43 % of a small population with concurrent pulmonary sarcoidosis [4]. SAPH most commonly presents with radiographically-advanced (Stage IV) pulmonary sarcoidosis [5]. In contrast to other forms of chronic lung disease-associated PH including idiopathic pulmonary fibrosis and chronic obstructive pulmonary disease where mild PH is most prevalent, SAPH typically manifests with more severe elevations in pulmonary pressures [6].

Pathophysiology

By convention, the World Health Organization (WHO) classification system has divided the various forms of PH into one of five classifications [7]. These groups include WHO classification group I (pulmonary arterial hypertension or PAH and its associated forms), group II (left-heart driven PH), group III (lung disease- and/or hypoxia-driven PH), group IV (chronic thromboembolic PH), and group V (unclear and/or multifactorial mechanisms). WHO classification V encompasses a variety of comorbid disease states associated with PH including pulmonary Langerhans cell histiocystosis, lymphangioleiomyomatosis, and sarcoidosis. The classification of SAPH as WHO group V or "multifactorial" PH speaks to the multiple potential pathologic mechanisms involved, and it can be argued that certain forms of SAPH can be labeled as multiple (if not all) WHO group classifications.

Because the majority SAPH have concurrent diffuse fibrotic lung disease, PH is typically thought to be secondary a combination of hypoxic vasoconstriction and capillary bed destruction. In addition, pulmonary vascular compression and distortion can occur at the level of alveolar vessels due to hyperinflation or at the proximal arteries/veins due to fibrosing mediastinitis or lymphadenopathy [8, 9]. However, between 32 and 50 % of SAPH can be present without associated pulmonary fibrosis, implicating alternative pathophysiologic mechanisms [10].

The pathologic hallmark of sarcoidosis is the presence of non-caseating granulomas, and granulomatous disease is thought to play a role in SAPH. Pulmonary venous granulomatous invasion is present in 65 % of pulmonary sarcoidosis cases, while pulmonary arterial involvement is present in 11 % [11, 12] (see Fig. 13.1). Consequently, occlusive arteriopathy and/or venopathy may develop, the relative

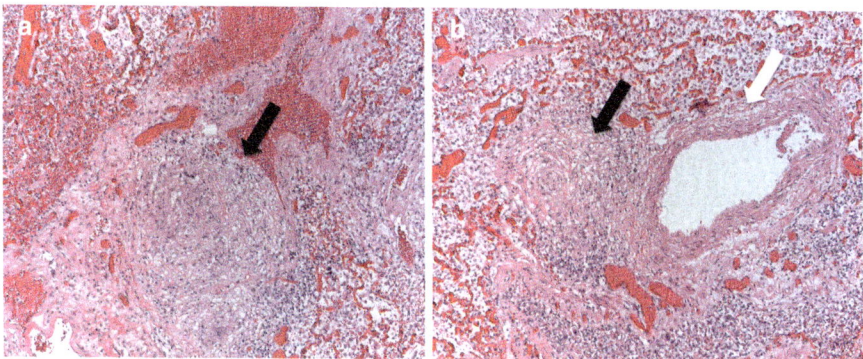

Fig. 13.1 Hematoxylin and eosin stained lung biopsy from a patient with sarcoidosis and severe pulmonary hypertension. (**a**) A granuloma (*black arrow*) in the wall of a pulmonary vein (**b**) A granuloma (*black arrow*) adjacent to the wall of a pulmonary artery (*white arrow*) (Images courtesy of Carlyne Cool, MD, National Jewish Health Pathology)

balance of which may dictate whether the hemodynamic profile resembles that of pulmonary arterial or pulmonary venous hypertension. Given the presence of pulmonary venous involvement, SAPH may have histopathologic and related hemodynamic features similar to pulmonary veno-occlusive disease [13–14].

The plexiform arteriopathy that is typically associated with PAH is a known but relatively rare finding in SAPH (see Fig. 13.2) [15]. Interestingly, there is growing recognition that sarcoidosis may increase the risk of thromboembolism [16, 17]. However, it has yet to be validated that this risk is associated with the development of SAPH from either pathophysiologic or epidemiologic studies.

Given the potential for comorbid cardiac involvement, SAPH due to left ventricular systolic or diastolic dysfunction remains an important consideration. A pulmonary artery occlusion pressure ≥15 mmHg was found to be present in 29 % in one SAPH series, suggesting left ventricular dysfunction as a contributor to PH [10].

Evaluation

An evaluation for SAPH should be considered whenever dyspnea appears to be disproportionate to the severity of the coexisting pulmonary sarcoidosis, when severe pulmonary sarcoidosis is present, or when right heart failure is present [18]. Echocardiography remains the mainstay of initial non-invasive evaluation for SAPH (see Fig. 13.3). An elevated right ventricular systolic pressure (RVSP) and/or features indicative of right heart remodeling including right ventricular enlargement, hypertrophy, and systolic dysfunction should raise the suspicion SAPH. However, reliance upon the use RVSP as an estimation of pulmonary artery systolic pressure can be misleading, particularly in patients with parenchymal lung disease [19, 20].

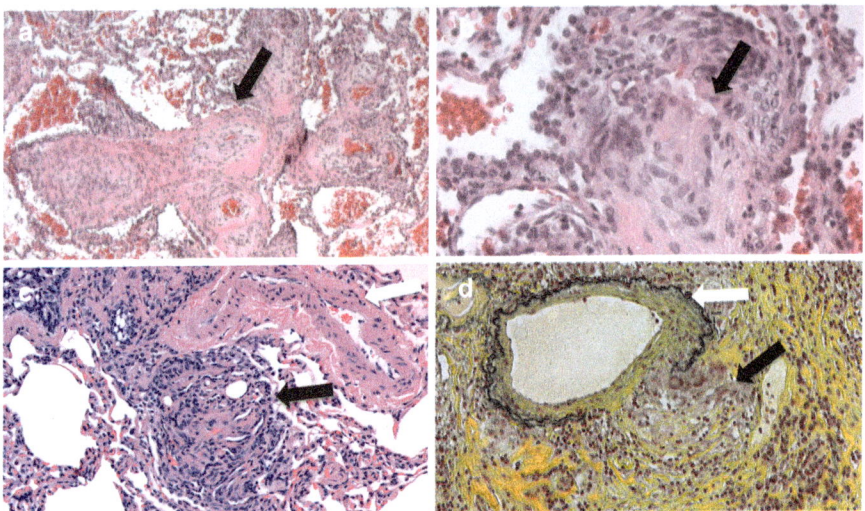

Fig. 13.2 Pulmonary biopsy specimens from: (**a**) A SAPH patient with plexiform arteriopathy demonstrating marked intimal thickening and hypertrophy (*black arrow*) (**b**) A SAPH patient with classic plexiform arteriopathy (*black arrow*) with intraluminal occlusion by endothelial and modified smooth muscle cells (**c**) A pulmonary hypertension patient with hematoxylin and eosin-stained biopsy demonstrating a plexiform lesion (*black arrow*) adjacent to a pulmonary arteriole (*white arrow*). Note the intravascular plug of endothelial cells forming multiple lamina. (**d**) A SAPH patient using pentachrome stain (*black* = elastic tissue, *yellow* = mature collagen, *blue-green* = immature collagen, *purple* = nuclei, *red* = smooth muscle/fibrin) demonstrating primarily mature collagen, nuclei, and elastic tissue. Note the granuloma i (*black arrow*) infiltrating the wall of the artery (*white arrow*) on the lower right (Images courtesy of Carlyne Cool, MD, National Jewish Health Pathology)

A multimodality testing approach should be incorporated into the initial SAPH evaluation (see Fig. 13.4). Electrocardiography may indicate the presence of right heart remodeling and corroborate echocardiographic findings. Chest radiographic staging of pulmonary sarcoidosis has utilized the Scadding score and stages patients from I to IV based upon the presence or absence of bilateral hilar lymphadenopathy, pulmonary infiltrates, fibrosis, and bullae [21]. The presence of an advanced Scadding stage should prompt consideration of the SAPH. The finding of ground glass attenuation, septal lines, and extrinsic compression of the pulmonary arteries by mediastinal adenopathy during chest computed tomography has been shown to be associated with SAPH [5]. Main pulmonary enlargement (PA) >29 mm or a ratio of the PA to aortic dimensions >1 has been proposed as a screening tool for PH, but its performance in SAPH has yet to be tested [22]. Surprisingly, neither spirometry, lung volumes, diffusion capacity, exertional hypoxemia, or 6 minute walk distance have proven to be reliably predictive of SAPH [3, 23, 24]. The relatively poor utility of these screening tests likely reflects not only the heterogeneous forms of SAPH but also the inherent limitations of each modality. Therefore, an optimal screening strategy should not rely upon individual test results but rather the composite of multiple tests as well as a symptoms, clinical course, and phenotype before determining whether to pursue diagnostic testing.

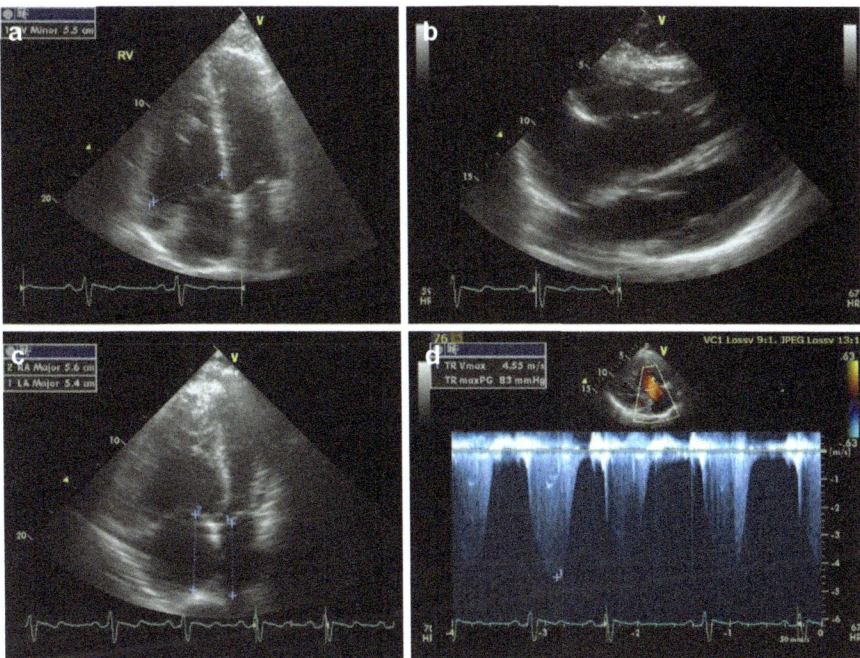

Fig. 13.3 Echocardiographic images from a 47 year old man with SAPH demonstrating significant right ventricular (*RV*) enlargement in (**a**) an apical four chamber view (RV major dimension 5.5 cm, normal <4.3 cm) and (**b**) a subcostal view. (**c**) An apical four chamber view showing mild right atrial (*RA*) enlargement (RA major dimension 5.6 cm, normal <5.4 cm) (**d**) A continuous wave Doppler tracing of tricuspid regurgitation showing a severely elevated right ventricular systolic pressure (83 mmHg, normal ≤35 mmHg)

Diagnosis

As with all forms of PH, the diagnosis of SAPH cannot be made noninvasively and requires a right heart catheterization to demonstrate an elevated mean pulmonary arterial pressure (mPAP) ≥25 mmHg [25]. This contrasts the diagnosis of PAH, which also requires elevated mPAP without an elevated left ventricular filling pressure as indicated by pulmonary capillary wedge pressure or left ventricular end diastolic pressure of ≤15 mmHg (see Fig. 13.5).

Treatment

In contrast to the well-established treatment algorithms for PAH, the optimal treatment approach to SAPH remains an area of controversy and active investigation. However, it is generally agreed upon that modifiable comorbid conditions that potentially contribute to SAPH should be identified and treated, including hypoxemia, obstructive sleep apnea, left ventricular systolic and/or diastolic dysfunction,

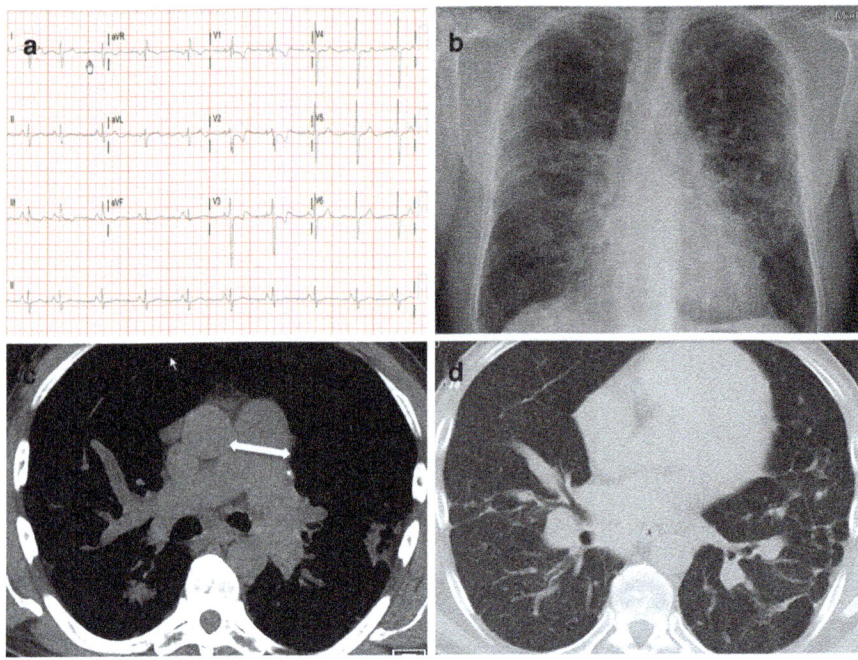

Fig. 13.4 Diagnostic testing from a 47 year old man with SAPH including: (**a**) an electrocardiogram demonstrating right ventricular hypertrophy and strain as well as right atrial enlargement (**b**) a chest x-ray showing mid and upper lung parahilar and peripheral reticulonodular opacities consistent with stage IV sarcoidosis (**c**) a chest computed tomogram (CT) demonstrating pulmonary arterial enlargement (3.9 cm, *white arrow*) (**d**) a chest CT showing diffuse lung fibrosis, consolidative opacities, and perihilar nodularity all consistent with pulmonary sarcoidosis

hypervolemia, and thromboembolic disease. Although corticosteroid therapy is theoretically appealing, its effect on pulmonary hemodynamics in small series has been highly variable and discrepant from improvement in pulmonary mechanics [26–28].

Pulmonary Vasodilators

Although the hemodynamic definition of PH is generally agreed upon, the hemodynamic phenotype that merits the use of targeted pulmonary vasodilator therapy is widely debated. As with other forms of non-WHO classification PH, there is an increasing movement to regard hemodynamically severe or "disproportionate" PH as distinct subtype that may behave like PAH and therefore benefit from drug therapy. When SAPH is viewed as a complication of chronic lung disease, severe PH has been defined as a mPAP ≥35 mmHg or mPAP ≥25 mmHg with low cardiac index (i.e., <2.0 l/min/m^2) [29]. Per the 5th World Symposium consensus guidelines, targeted pulmonary vasodilator therapy should be considered on a compassionate basis for this subpopulation with thorough monitoring of gas exchange and inclusion in prospective registries.

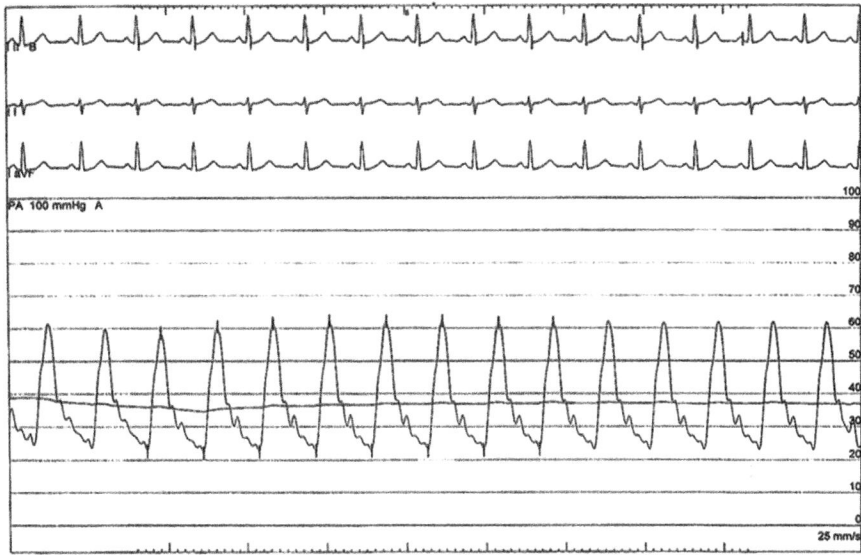

Fig. 13.5 Pulmonary artery pressure waveform from a right heart catheterization in 47 year old man with stage IV pulmonary sarcoidosis and SAPH. The pulmonary artery pressure was 63/23 mmHg (mean 37 mmHg), pulmonary capillary wedge pressure 14 mmHg, and pulmonary vascular resistance of 6 Woods units

Although a growing body of evidence suggests a potential benefit of PAH-specific pharmacologic therapies in SAPH, this literature is limited to small controlled studies, and more commonly, case series. In a recent small, randomized study comparing the endothelin receptor antagonist bosentan to placebo in SAPH, bosentan significantly decreased mean pulmonary artery pressure and pulmonary vascular resistance after 16 weeks of therapy without improving 6 min walk distance [30]. Similarly, in a retrospective study of 12 SAPH patients with end-stage pulmonary sarcoidosis, sildenafil failed to improve 6 min walk distance but did reduce both mPAP and PVR while increasing cardiac index [31]. Prostacyclin therapy has also demonstrated benefit, albeit in very small case series. Use of inhaled iloprost in SAPH improved pulmonary hemodynamics, 6 min walk distance, and quality of life in a subset of patients [32]. However, use of these agents should be tempered by limited data supporting their use as well as concerns that pulmonary vasodilator therapy may precipitate ventilation/perfusion mismatch, particularly in SAPH patients with significant hypoxemia and/or pulmonary fibrosis.

Transplant

The critical role PH plays in the outcomes of sarcoidosis is reflected in the International Society of Heart Lung Transplant consensus guidelines for lung transplantation. Referral for lung transplant evaluation is recommended in patients with

New York Heart Association Functional Class III or IV symptom, hypoxemia at rest, right atrial pressure of 15 mmHg, or PH [33].

Prognosis

SAPH patients are more likely to experience debilitating dyspnea, exercise intolerance, and reduced functional capacity [34, 35]. In a population with pulmonary sarcoidosis awaiting lung transplant, the presence of PH predicted a poor prognosis [36, 37]. The estimated 5-year survival for SAPH is only 59 %. Little is known about the impact of pulmonary vasodilator therapy on mortality in SAPH.

Conclusion

SAPH represents a heterogeneous set of diseases which challenges the current framework for our understanding the pathophysiologic origins of PH. Although considerable progress has been made towards elucidating pathologic mechanisms, clinical phenotypes, and treatment selection, significant knowledge gaps persist. Similar to other forms of non-PAH PH, the optimal treatment approach to SAPH remains essentially unknown. Because SAPH may share certain pathophysiologic mechanisms with other forms of PH, ongoing investigations into hypoxia/chronic lung disease-associated PH and pulmonary venous hypertension may better inform our understanding of SAPH. However, improving outcomes in SAPH will ultimately require prospective, blinded studies that recognize the unique nature of sarcoidosis and its multitude of clinical phenotypes, each of which may require a phenotype-specific approach. In the meantime, SAPH is likely to remain a challenging problem for the patient and clinician alike.

Pearls
1. Sarcoidosis associated pulmonary hypertension (SAPH) most commonly, though not always, presents with radiographically-advanced pulmonary sarcoidosis.
2. SAPH confers a poor prognosis and is associated with a greater likelihood of experiencing debilitating dyspnea, exercise intolerance, and reduced functional capacity.
3. Similar to other forms of PH, the diagnosis of SAPH requires a right heart catheterization to demonstrate a mean pulmonary artery pressure of 25 mmHg or higher.
4. Although there is a growing body of evidence to suggest possible benefit of PAH-specific therapies in SAPH, there are no currently FDA approved medications for SAPH.

References

1. Baughman RP, Culver DA, Judson MA. A concise review of pulmonary sarcoidosis. Am J Respir Crit Care Med. 2011;183:573–81.
2. Handa T, Nagai S, Miki S, et al. Incidence of pulmonary hypertension and its clinical relevance in patients with sarcoidosis. Chest. 2006;129:1246–52.
3. Bourbonnais JM, Samavati L. Clinical predictors of pulmonary hypertension in sarcoidosis. Eur Respir J. 2008;32:296–302.
4. Gluskowski J, Hawrylkiewicz I, Zych D, et al. Pulmonary haemodynamics at rest and during exercise in patients with sarcoidosis. Respiration. 1984;46:26–32.
5. Nunes H, Humbert M, Capron F, et al. Pulmonary hypertension associated with sarcoidosis: mechanisms, haemodynamics and prognosis. Thorax. 2006;61:68–74.
6. Nathan SD, Hassoun PM. Pulmonary hypertension due to lung disease and/or hypoxia. Clin Chest Med. 2013;34:695–705.
7. Simonneau G, Gatzoulis MA, Adatia I, Celermajer D, Denton C, Ghofrani A, Gomez Sanchez MA, Krishna Kumar R, Landzberg M, Machado RF, Olschewski H, Robbins IM, Souza R. Updated clinical classification of pulmonary hypertension. J Am Coll Cardiol. 2013;62:D34–41.
8. Berry DF, Buccigrossi D, Peabody J, et al. Pulmonary vascular occlusion and fibrosing mediastinitis. Chest. 1986;89:296–301.
9. Ferguson ME, Cabalka AK, Cetta F, et al. Results of intravascular stent placement for fibrosing mediastinitis. Congenit Heart Dis. 2010;5:124–33.
10. Baughman RP, Engel PJ, Taylor L, Lower EE. Survival in sarcoidosis associated pulmonary hypertension: the importance of hemodynamic evaluation. Chest. 2010;138:1078–85.
11. Rosen Y, Moon S, Huang CT, et al. Granulomatous pulmonary angiitis in sarcoidosis. Arch Pathol Lab Med. 1977;101:170.
12. Takemura T, Matsui Y, Oritsu M, et al. Pulmonary vascular involvement in sarcoidosis: granulomatous angiitis and microangiopathy in transbronchial lung biopsies. Virchows Arch A Pathol Anat Histopathol. 1991;418:361.
13. Hoffstein V, Ranganathan N, Mullen JB. Sarcoidosis simulating pulmonary venoocclusive disease. Am Rev Respir Dis. 1986;134:809–11.
14. Jones RM, Dawson A, Jenkins GH, Nicholson AG, Hansell DM, Harrison NK. Sarcoidosis related pulmonary veno-occlusive disease presenting with recurrent haemoptysis. Eur Respir J. 2009;34:517–20.
15. Tayal S, Voelkel NF, Rai PR, et al. Sarcoidois and pulmonary hypertension–a case report. Eur J Med Res. 2006;11:194–7.
16. Swigris JJ, Olson AL, Huie TJ, et al. Increased risk of pulmonary embolism among US decedents with sarcoidosis from 1988 to 2007. Chest. 2011;140:1261–6.
17. Crawshaw AP, Wotton CJ, Yeates DG, Goldacre MJ, Ho LP. Evidence for association between sarcoidosis and pulmonary embolism from 35-year record linkage study. Thorax. 2011;66:447–8.
18. Nunes H, Uzunhan Y, Freynet O, Humbert M, Brillet PY, Kambouchner M, Valeyre D. Pulmonary hypertension complicating sarcoidosis. Presse Med. 2012;41:e303–16.
19. Arcasoy SM, Christie JD, Ferrari VA, et al. Echocardiographic assessment of pulmonary hypertension in patients with advanced lung disease. Am J Respir Crit Care Med. 2003;167:735–40.
20. Fisher MR, Criner GJ, Fishman AP, et al. Estimating pulmonary artery pressures by echocardiography in patients with emphysema. Eur Respir J. 2007;30:914–21.
21. Scadding JG. Prognosis of intrathoracic sarcoidosis in England: a review of 136 cases after five years' observation. BMJ. 1961;2:1165–72.
22. Corson N, Armato 3rd SG, Labby ZE, Straus C, Starkey A, Gomberg-Maitland M. CT-based pulmonary artery measurements for the assessment of pulmonary hypertension. Acad Radiol. 2014;21:523–30.

23. Shorr AF, Helman DL, Davies DB, Nathan SD. Pulmonary hypertension in advanced sarcoidosis: epidemiology and clinical characteristics. Eur Respir J. 2005;25:783–8.
24. Sulica R, Teirstein AS, Kakarla S, Nemani N, Behnegar A, Padilla ML. Distinctive clinical, radiographic, and functional characteristics of patients with sarcoidosis-related pulmonary hypertension. Chest. 2005;128:1483–9.
25. Hoeper MM, Bogaard HJ, Condliffe R, Frantz R, Khanna D, Kurzyna M, Langleben D, Manes A, Satoh T, Torres F, Wilkins MR, Badesch DB. Definitions and diagnosis of pulmonary hypertension. J Am Coll Cardiol. 2013;62:D42–50.
26. Rodman DM, Lindenfeld J. Successful treatment of sarcoidosis-associated pulmonary hypertension with corticosteroids. Chest. 1990;97:500–2.
27. Toonkel RL, Borczuk AC, Pearson GD, Horn EM, Thomashow BM. Sarcoidosis-associated fibrosing mediastinitis with resultant pulmonary hypertension: a case report and review of the literature. Respiration. 2010;79:341–5.
28. Gluskowski J, Hawrylkiewicz I, Zych D, Zieliński J. Effects of corticosteroid treatment on pulmonary haemodynamics in patients with sarcoidosis. Eur Respir J. 1990;3:403–7.
29. Seeger W, Adir Y, Barberà JA, Champion H, Coghlan JG, Cottin V, De Marco T, Galiè N, Ghio S, Gibbs S, Martinez FJ, Semigran MJ, Simonneau G, Wells AU, Vachiéry JL. Pulmonary hypertension in chronic lung diseases. J Am Coll Cardiol. 2013;62:D109–16.
30. Baughman RP, Culver DA, Cordova FC, Padilla M, Gibson KF, Lower EE, Engel PJ. Bosentan for sarcoidosis-associated pulmonary hypertension: a double-blind placebo controlled randomized trial. Chest. 2014;145:810–7.
31. Milman N, Burton CM, Iversen M, et al. Pulmonary hypertension in end-stage pulmonary sarcoidosis: therapeutic effect of sildenafil? J Heart Lung Transplant. 2008;75:329–34.
32. Baughman RP, Judson MA, Lower EE, et al. Inhaled iloprost for sarcoidosis associated pulmonary hypertension. Sarcoidosis Vasc Diffuse Lung Dis. 2009;26:110–20.
33. Orens JB, Estenne M, Arcasoy S, Conte JV, Corris P, Egan JJ, Egan T, Keshavjee S, Knoop C, Kotloff R, Martinez FJ, Nathan S, Palmer S, Patterson A, Singer L, Snell G, Studer S, Vachiery JL, Glanville AR, Pulmonary Scientific Council of the International Society for Heart and Lung Transplantation. International guidelines for the selection of lung transplant candidates: 2006 update – a consensus report from the Pulmonary Scientific Council of the International Society for Heart and Lung Transplantation. J Heart Lung Transplant. 2006;25:745–55.
34. Baughman RP, Engel PJ, Meyer CA, Barrett AB, Lower EE. Pulmonary hypertension in sarcoidosis. Sarcoidosis Vasc Diffuse Lung Dis. 2006;23:108–16.
35. Baughman RP, Sparkman BK, Lower EE. Six minute walk test and health status assessment in sarcoidosis. Chest. 2007;132:207–13.
36. Neville E, Walker AN, James DG. Prognostic factors predicting the outcome of sarcoidosis: an analysis of 818 patients. Q J Med. 1983;52:525–33.
37. Shorr AF, Davies DB, Nathan SD. Predicting mortality in patients with sarcoidosis awaiting lung transplantation. Chest. 2003;124:922–8.

Chapter 14
Cases in Cardiac Sarcoidosis

Andrew M. Freeman, Howard D. Weinbeger, Darlene Kim, Brett Fenster, Joyce D. Schroeder, Nabeel Y. Hamzeh, William H. Sauer, Matthew M. Zipse, Divya Patel, Ron Blankstein, Sharmila Dorbala, Edward J. Miller, Neal K. Lakdawala, and Garrick C. Stewart

Abstract Cardiac sarcoidosis continues to be a very challenging diagnosis and can prove to be even more challenging to manage. In this case series, the authors will walk the reader through difficult cases in the management of real-life cases of sarcoidosis with cardiac involvement. Imaging results, catheterization and biopsy results, clinical scenarios, and pitfalls in the care of these patients will be reviewed through case examples with summaries of key points.

A.M. Freeman, MD, FACC, FACP (✉) • H.D. Weinbeger, MD, FACC, FACP
D. Kim, MD, FACC • B. Fenster, MD, FACC, FACP, FASE
Division of Cardiology, Department of Medicine, National Jewish Health,
1400 Jackson St., Denver, CO 80206, USA
e-mail: freemana@njhealth.org; weinbergerh@njhealth.org; kimd@njhealth.org; fensterb@njhealth.org

J.D. Schroeder, MD
Department of Radiology, University of Colorado,
Adjoint Associate Professor, Aurora, CO, USA
e-mail: joyce.schroeder@stanfordalumni.org

N.Y. Hamzeh, MD
Division of Environmental and Occupational Health Sciences, Department of Medicine,
National Jewish Health, 1400 Jackson St., Denver, CO 80206, USA

Division of Pulmonary and Critical Care Sciences, Department of Medicine,
University of Colorado Hospital, 12401 East 17th Avenue, Aurora, CO, USA
e-mail: hamzehn@njhealth.org

W.H. Sauer, MD • M.M. Zipse, MD
Section of Cardiac Electrophysiology, Division of Cardiology, University of Colorado
Hospital, 12401 East 17th Avenue, B136, Aurora, CO 80045, USA
e-mail: william.sauer@ucdenver.edu; Matthew.Zipse@ucdenver.edu

D. Patel, DO
Division of Pulmonary and Critical Care Sciences, Department of Medicine, University of
Colorado Hospital, 12401 East 17th Avenue, Aurora, CO, USA
e-mail: divcpatel@gmail.com

R. Blankstein, MD, FACC • S. Dorbala, MD, MPH
Non-invasive Cardiovascular Imaging Program, Department of Medicine (Cardiovascular Division) and Department of Radiology, Brigham and Women's Hospital, Harvard Medical School, Shapiro Room 5096 75 Francis Street, Boston, MA 02115, USA
e-mail: rblankstein@partners.org; sdorbala@partners.org

E.J. Miller, MD, PhD
Section of Cardiovascular Medicine, Boston University School of Medicine,
88 E. Newton Street, Boston, MA 02118, USA
e-mail: ejmiller@bu.edu

N.K. Lakdawala, MD • G.C. Stewart, MD
Cardiovascular Medicine, Boston University School of Medicine,
75 Francis Street, Boston, MA 02118, USA
e-mail: nlakdawala@partners.org; gcstewart@partners.org

Cardiac Sarcoidosis Clinical Vignette #1

A 44-year-old male with a history of hypertension and elevated cholesterol presented to the local emergency department after a brief episode of syncope. He states that he was getting ready for work, "passed out" and fell onto his bed. He thinks he was only out for a few seconds. He denied any palpitations, chest pain, tightness or discomfort, or other symptoms at that time. He had experienced several episodes of light headedness and near syncope for several days before his syncopal episode and had noted some "chest congestion" and cough over the preceding 2 months. An ECG in the emergency department demonstrated complete heart block. He was evaluated by a local cardiologist and had a permanent pacemaker implanted for complete heart block (see Fig. 14.1). Further evaluation at that time included an

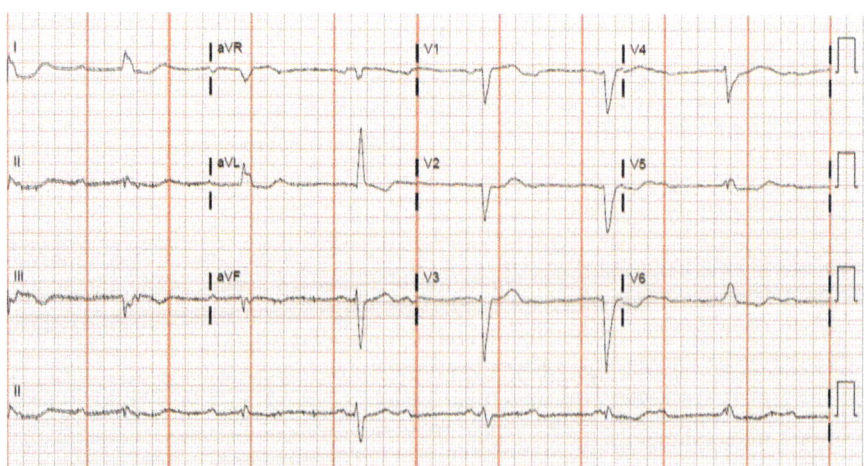

Fig. 14.1 Electrocardiogram (*ECG*) demonstrating complete heart block

echocardiogram which revealed moderately to severely reduced left ventricular systolic function with a LVEF of approximately 30 %, and coronary angiography with no obstructive coronary artery disease. He was referred for endomyocardial biopsy a few weeks after his initial presentation, given his non-ischemic cardiomyopathy and complete heart block. His right ventricular endomyocardial biopsy showed multifocal giant cell noncaseating granulomas consistent with sarcoidosis.

After the endomyocardial biopsy results returned indicating myocardial sarcoidosis, he was started on prednisone 60 mg daily which was tapered down to 40 mg daily over 2 months, and he was referred to National Jewish Health for evaluation and management of his sarcoidosis. Evaluation at that time included a signal averaged ECG which was abnormal, and an echocardiogram showing LV enlargement with LVEF of 38 %, stage II LV diastolic dysfunction, biatrial enlargement and pacemaker wire in the right ventricle. Appropriate heart failure beta blocker and angiotensin converting enzyme inhibitor therapies had previously been initiated, and were up-titrated. It was recommended that the patient have his pacemaker upgraded to an ICD, which was done by his local cardiologist's office.

Cardiac Sarcoidosis Clinical Vignette #2

A 40-year old woman with a history of progressive shortness of breath and palpitations for 3 months presented with syncope. She was found to have a reduced left ventricular ejection fraction of 40–45 % with inferoseptal hypokinesis and mild right ventricular enlargement. ECG demonstrated an incomplete right bundle branch block. Coronary angiography demonstrated no significant coronary artery disease, and chest radiograph demonstrated small left-sided pleural effusion and mild pulmonary vascular congestion.

Holter monitoring demonstrated runs of non-sustained left bundle branch morphology ventricular tachycardia (Fig. 14.2). The diagnosis of arrhythmogenic right ventricular cardiomyopathy was considered. She underwent a cardiac MRI and was found with delayed gadolinium enhancement of the inferoseptal wall and normal right ventricular size and function. Chest CT demonstrated no hilar lymphadenopathy. Endomyocardial biopsy was then performed, with attempts to obtain samples in the region of delayed gadolinium enhancement and guided by electroanatomic mapping (Fig. 14.3). Pathology demonstrated non-caseating granulomas, and a diagnosis of sarcoidosis was confirmed.

She was started on high dose corticosteroids. The patient had a recurrent syncopal episode, and ECG at that time demonstrated Mobitz type 2 second-degree AV block (Fig. 14.4). An ICD/pacemaker was implanted as a result. Three months later, repeat echocardiogram showed improvement in ejection fraction to 55–60 %, and as she had no recurrent arrhythmia or heart block on repeat cardiac monitoring, a slow taper in steroid dose was started.

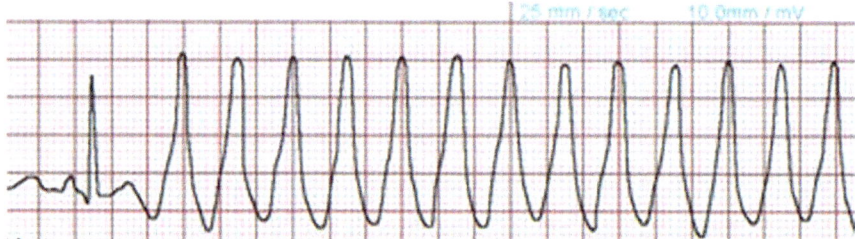

Fig. 14.2 Rhythm strip demonstrating a run of non-sustained ventricular tachycardia

14 Cases in Cardiac Sarcoidosis

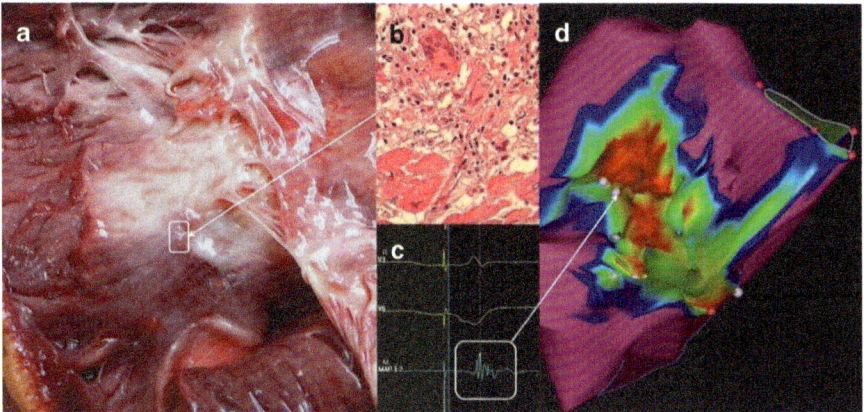

Fig. 14.3 (**a**) and (**b**) Representative examples of gross granulomatous myocardial scarring and microscopic noncaseating granuloma infiltrating myocardium (**c**) Low-amplitude intracardiac electrogram at an involved site (**d**) Electroanatomic map demonstrating reduced voltage corresponding to areas of myocardial scar caused by sarcoid granuloma

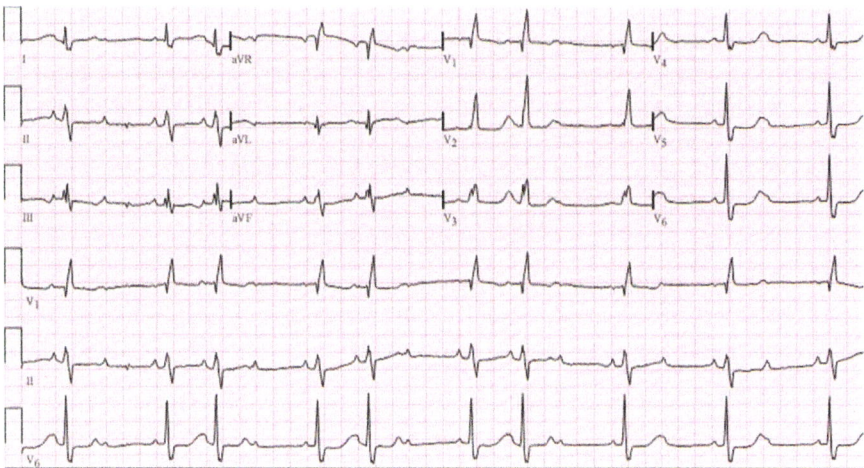

Fig. 14.4 ECG at that time demonstrated Mobitz type 2 second-degree AV block

Cardiac Sarcoidosis Clinical Vignette #3

The patient is a 60-year-old white man with a history of biopsy-proven pulmonary sarcoidosis from 5 years ago, which initially manifested with shortness of breath and pleurisy that resulted in chest imaging leading to biopsy. He had a history of pericardial effusion with his bout of pleurisy that was self-limited and resolved on its own. He had a past medical history significant for dyslipidemia, nephrolithiasis, and borderline enlarged aorta, and incidental coronary calcification seen on chest computed tomography (CT). He was being treated by a colleague in pulmonary medicine with hydroxychloroquine and prednisone intermittently with some success.

His family history was significant for extensive for coronary disease. His mother died at age 47 from lymphoma/cancer. A maternal grandfather died at age 58 from a myocardial infarction, two maternal uncles were affected by heart disease; one died at age 70 from a myocardial infarction and one is alive at age 83 with his first myocardial infarction in his 60s. His father was deceased, dying at age 69 from a myocardial infarction, and the patient's older brother was a questionable blue baby with "congenital heart disease", likely a significant atrial septal defect or ventricular septal defect per the description – the patient wasn't entirely sure.

The patient's major complaint was shortness of breath resulting in limitations in some of the things he enjoyed doing, in addition to chest tightness he occasionally noticed when going to the gym to exercise. It would come on with activity and resolve with rest usually within 4–5 min. These symptoms persisted despite prednisone and hydroxychloroquine.

His ECG in the office showed first-degree atrio-ventricular (AV) block and non-specific ST-T wave abnormalities (Fig. 14.5).

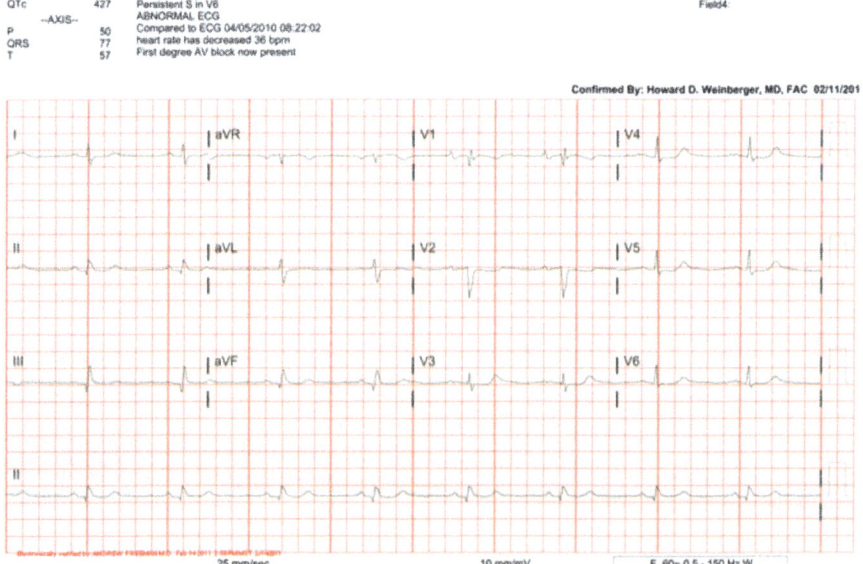

Fig. 14.5 ECG demonstrating first degree AV block

His cardiac exam, much to his physicians' surprise, was largely unremarkable.

As a result of his symptoms, a stress test was arranged which demonstrated transient ST elevations in the inferior leads. In addition, in recovery he had ST depressions, which persisted for several minutes and then resolved with slower heart rates. These findings resulted in the patient being sent, by ambulance, to the nearest hospital where a coronary angiogram and catheterization were performed.

The catheterization showed a 50–70 % left anterior descending (LAD) artery stenosis, his second obtuse marginal (OM2) artery with a 70 % occlusion, his first obtuse marginal (OM1) artery with an 80 % occlusion, the left circumflex (LCx) artery distal total occlusion and a chronic total occlusion of his right coronary artery (RCA), receiving collaterals from the LCx.

Interestingly, his echocardiogram remained normal with preserved left ventricular ejection fraction, no pericardial effusion, and normal right ventricular function with normal estimated pulmonary artery systolic pressures.

His signal averaged ECG, however, remained abnormal in three out of three domains throughout his therapy (Fig. 14.6).

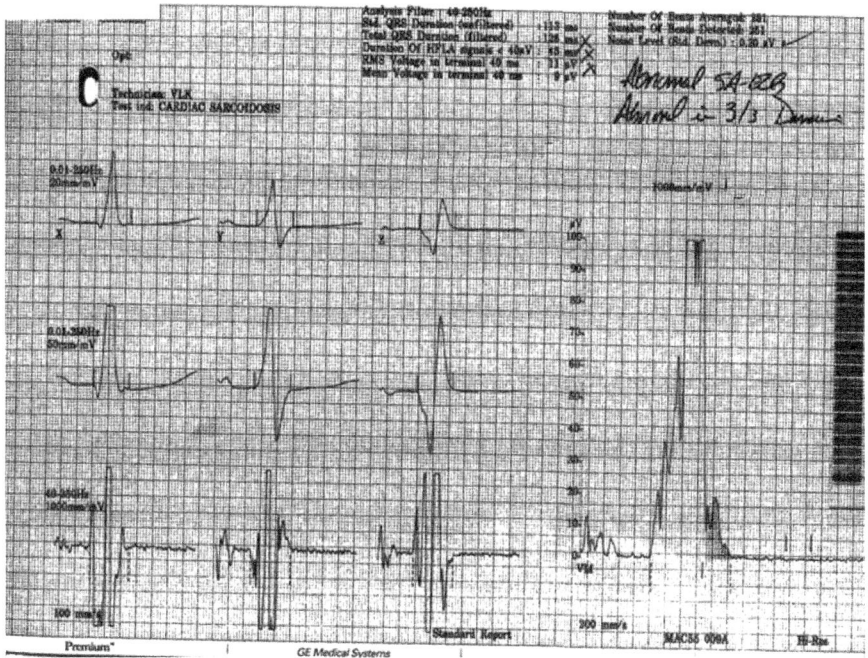

Fig. 14.6 Signal averaged ECG demonstrating three out of three abnormal domains

Advanced imaging with cardiac MRI was surprisingly without areas of delayed contrast hyperenhancement, though 18-FDG myocardial PET did show some patchiness suggesting areas of inflammation (Fig. 14.7, 14.8, and 14.9).

At this point, the decision was made to perform coronary artery bypass grafting (CABG), but because of a densely adherent pericardium, only a left internal mam-

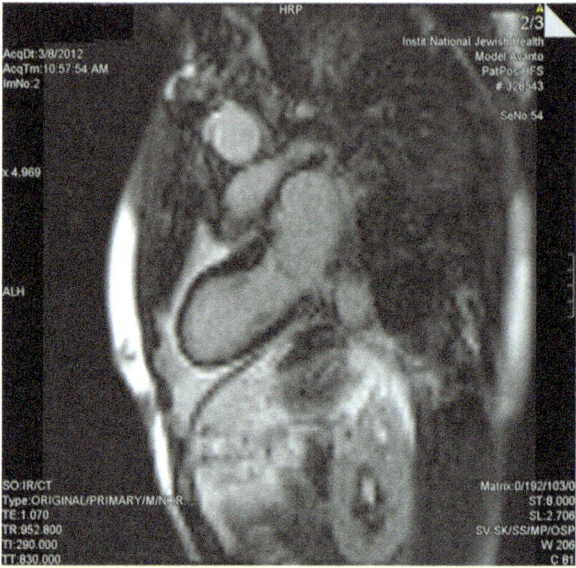

Fig. 14.7 Cardiac MRI delayed contrast enhancement image (vertical long axis) demonstrating no clear focal enhancement

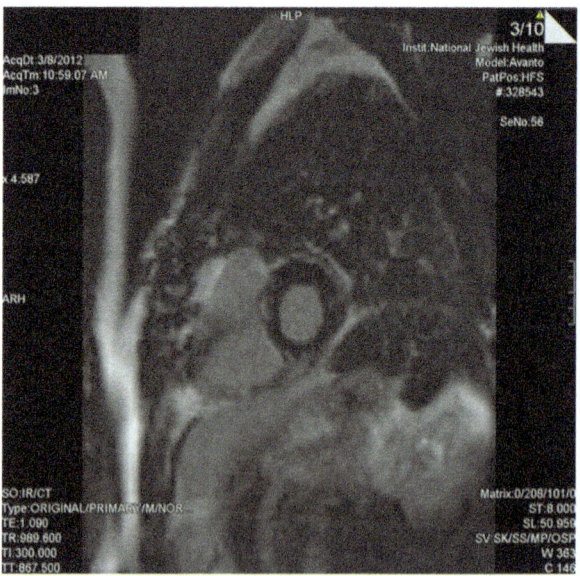

Fig. 14.8 Cardiac MRI delayed contrast enhancement image (short axis) demonstrating no clear focal enhancement

Fig. 14.9 18-FDG myocardial PET demonstrating patchy on diffuse hypermetabolic activity suggesting active inflammation. Note myocardial and likely pericardial involvement

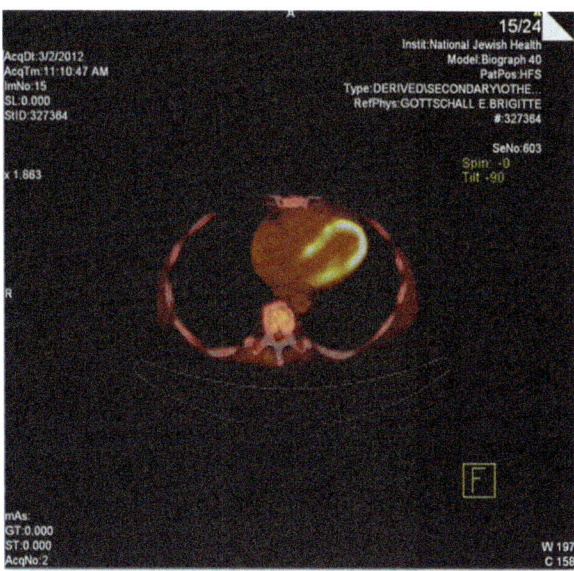

mary artery (LIMA) to left anterior descending (LAD) artery bypass could be performed. Subsequently, he received a stent to his left circumflex (LCx) artery which completed the revascularization as best as was possible.

These interventions resulted in him feeling better, but shortly after surgery he developed volume overload and required intensive diuresis.

Just when things appeared to be settling down for this patient, he had an episode of supraventricular tachycardia (SVT) with heart rates >160 bpm resulting in another emergency room visit with a diagnosis of atrioventricular nodal re-entrant tachycardia (AVNRT). He underwent an ablation (and a concurrent right ventricular voltage map and programmed electrical stimulation study which was negative for inducible ventricular tachycardia).

Once all of the above issues were settled, the patient went on vacation to Florida (USA) and played golf for an extended period of time in the heat of the Florida summer. As he was also on a statin with his intensive coronary disease, his urine turned red in color prompting another emergency room visit for mild rhabdomyolysis that resolved with hydration and discontinuation of the statin.

Eventually, the patient's condition returned to normal and he has been successful at improving his lifestyle, diet, and exercise and has tolerated low dose statins without much trouble.

Interesting Points

1. Cardiac sarcoidosis can present with normal heart function, but still have pericardial involvement with rhythm disturbances, including first degree AV block.
2. Cardiac MRI did not show evidence for scarring with delayed contrast hyperenhancement, but, 18-FDG myocardial PET did show patchy inflammation on top of overall inflammation.
3. While an echocardiogram did not show any abnormalities, an abnormal signal-averaged ECG raised a strong possibility for cardiac sarcoidosis early on in the case.
4. Pericardial involvement is uncommon even in the presence of extensive myocardial infiltration. It is observed in fewer than 10 % of patients with cardiac sarcoidosis, and these patients usually remain asymptomatic [1].
5. Small pericardial effusions detected by echocardiography were found in 19 % of patients with sarcoidosis [2].

Cardiac Sarcoidosis Clinical Vignette #4

A 75 year old Japanese woman diagnosed with sarcoidosis 21 years previously with skin and eye involvement treated with local and topical steroids. Two years after her diagnosis of sarcoidosis, she suffered a sudden cardiac arrest event but was successfully resuscitated by emergency medical services. An automated implantable cardioverter defibrillator (AICD) was implanted and she has been well since then.

Two years previously, she began to complain of a vibrating and fluttering sensation in her chest and interrogation of her AICD revealed several appropriate antitachycardia pacing interventions by her AICD for ventricular tachycardia in the past 2–3 months. She was subsequently referred to our granuloma clinic for further assessment and management of potential active sarcoidosis myocarditis. Her cardiac medications at the time of presentation included sotalol, losartan and aspirin. Her initial physical exam revealed stable vital signs and overall unremarkable physical exam.

Initial workup included the following:

- Twelve lead ECG: Sinus rhythm, rate of 67, normal axis, interventricular conduction delay with nonspecific ST and T-wave changes.
- Echocardiogram: Normal left ventricular size and wall thickness with mildly reduced overall systolic function, estimated left ventricular ejection fraction 40–50 %. Basal infero-septal and posterior wall thinning with akinesis.

She was subsequently started on prednisone at 20 mg daily for 2 months followed by a slow tapering schedule over the next 4 months, and concomitant oral methotrexate starting at 7.5 mg weekly up-titrated gradually to a maintenance dose of 15 mg weekly with folic acid supplementation on a daily basis. Cardiac magnetic resonance imaging could not be performed due to the AICD.

On follow up and since starting her immunosuppressive regimens, she has had one to two arrhythmic events that did not require any intervention by her AICD. Her echocardiogram remained stable without change in her LV function, LVEF or wall motion abnormalities. She is currently maintained on methotrexate 15 mg weekly, has not required any interventions from her AICD and has not required any ablation procedures. Her cardiac medications remained stable throughout her course.

Interesting Points

This case highlights the potential causes of new or worsening arrhythmias in patients with known cardiac sarcoidosis. New or worsening arrhythmias can develop either due to active granulomatous myocarditis or due to scar formation (new or pre-existing). Arrhythmias due to active myocarditis are usually responsive to immunosuppressive therapy and the preferred agent is corticosteroids due to its rapid onset. The ideal dose is not exactly known but based on available literature [3] and expert consensus [4] a dose of 30–40 mg of prednisone daily (or equivalent) is usually recommended. Our case demonstrated a rapid improvement and resolution of her arrhythmias with immunosuppressive therapy and she did not require ablative therapy.

Cardiac Sarcoidosis Clinical Vignette #5

In this case report, a patient with cardiac sarcoidosis was successfully treated with catheter ablation for the treatment of ventricular arrhythmias refractory to anti-arrhythmic and immunosuppressive therapy.

A 58 year-old man with a prior history of cardiac sarcoidosis with preserved ejection fraction presented with frequent episodes of syncope and near syncope. While on telemetry monitoring, spontaneous salvos of non-sustained ventricular tachycardia (NSVT) were observed corresponding to symptoms of light-headedness (Fig. 14.10). The patient was given amiodarone and empiric immunosuppression with incomplete suppression of the spontaneous arrhythmias. Because of the frequency of the symptomatic ventricular arrhythmias refractory to medical therapy, catheter ablation was performed.

The initial endocardial voltage map revealed a small amount of right and left ventricular scar (Fig. 14.11). Activation mapping of frequent premature ventricular contractions (PVCs) that matched the morphology of the spontaneous NSVT revealed an area of diffuse activation at the basal free wall of the right ventricle. The morphological characteristics of the electrogram (predominant early far-field

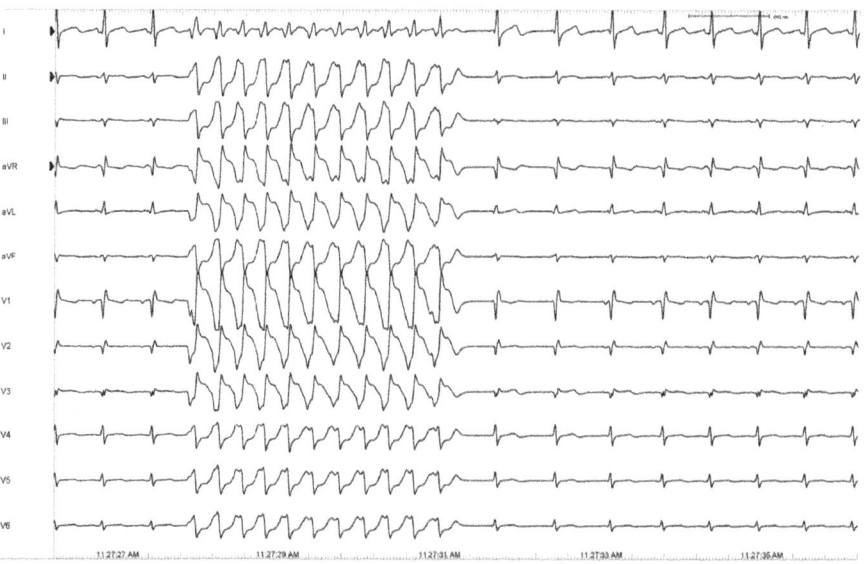

Fig. 14.10 Twelve-lead electrocardiogram of spontaneous and rapid non-sustained ventricular tachycardia

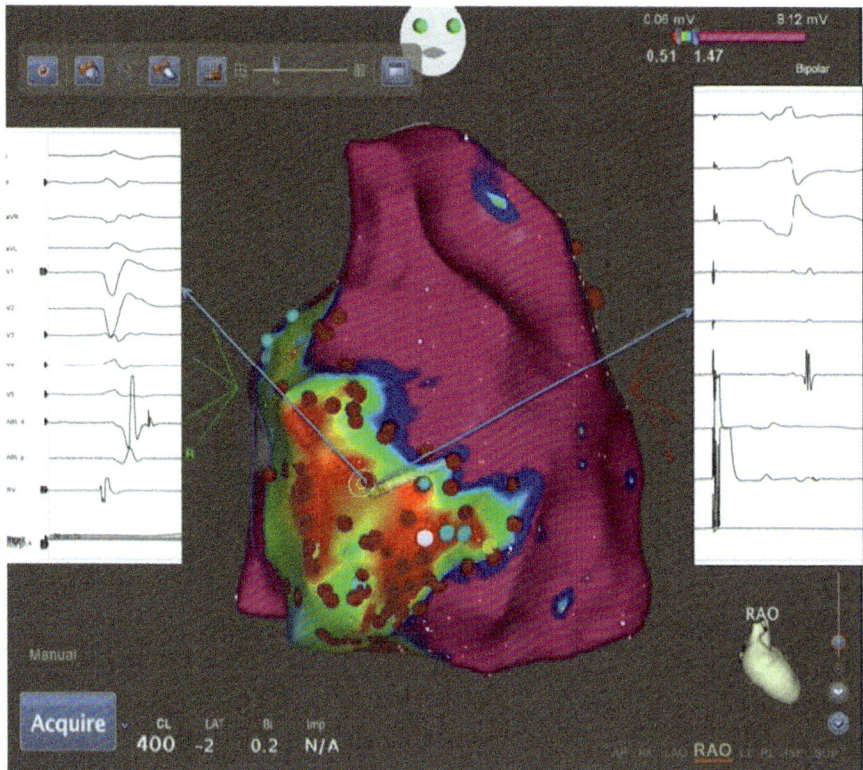

Fig. 14.11 Electroanatomical map of the epicardial right ventricle with a sample of a recorded electrogram in the borderzone of scar identifying the presence of near field electrical signals after the inscription of the QRS complex (late potential)

electrogram) with a diffuse early endocardial activation indicated an epicardial site of origin for the VT. Therefore epicardial access was obtained for continued mapping of the arrhythmogenic tissue.

During sinus rhythm, the electroanatomical voltage map on the epicardial surface revealed a large heterogeneous area of reduced voltage at the basal free wall immediately opposite to the sites of early activation on the endocardial surface. Upon induction of general anesthesia and access to the epicardium, the tachycardia was no longer observed, therefore a strategy of pacemapping with affected regions of scar was used to identify ablation targets. Ablation of all abnormal signals within the hertergenous scar yielding perfect or near-perfect pacemaps was performed.

Following ablation, the patient had no further ectopy or ventricular tachycardia and has been free of any ventricular arrhythmia over the course of 3 years of follow-up off of immunosuppressive and anti-arrhythmic drug therapy.

Interesting Points

This case is illustrative of several important and unique characteristics of sarcoidosis related ventricular arrhythmias. The mechanism of the ventricular arrhythmia was proven to be related to the heterogeneous scar identified on the epicardial surface. Only after epicardial access was obtained, could this scar be revealed and appropriately targeted for ablation. Prior studies [5, 6] evaluating VT related to cardiac sarcoidosis have noted epicardial involvement, and thus this case demonstrates the need to evaluate this possibility for successful ablation.

An interesting aspect of this case was the inability to control the ventricular arrhythmias with pharmacologic therapy. Several investigators have reported cases where immunosuppression was effective in suppressing ventricular arrhythmias in cardiac sarcoidoisis patients with evidence of active inflammation [7]. In this case, the use of anti-arrhythmic and immunosuppressive agents was not effective in controlling symptoms related to the arrhythmia.

Finally, ablation attempts for treatment of ventricular arrhythmias related to cardiac sarcoidosis are often not successful due to the wide distribution of scar in the endocardium, epicardium, and mid-myocardium as well as an unpredictable progression of the sarcoidosis itself [8]. In this particular case, a single region was identified as an ablation target possibly increasing the chances for long-term success.

In summary, this case demonstrates how ablation can be required for successful management of drug-refractory symptomatic ventricular arrhythmias related to cardiac sarcoidosis.

Cardiac Sarcoidosis Clinical Vignette #6

As described in Chap. 9, patients with cardiac sarcoidosis can present with varying degrees of heart block due to septal inflammation and scarring. While long term scarring of the basal septum resulting in heart block is irreversible, if the mechanism of heart block is instead inflammation related to granulomatous infiltration that has not yet resulted in scar, immunosuppression and/or corticosteroids can potentially recover atrioventricular conduction.

A 43 year old man with cardiac sarcoidosis originally presented with symptomatic second degree AV block Type 2 requiring the implantation of a permanent pacemaker in 2004. This device was later upgraded to a dual chamber implantable cardioverter-defibrillator (ICD) in 2006 because of concern for sudden death risk due to progression of cardiac sarcoidosis. In addition to worsening left ventricular dysfunction, the patient progressed to complete heart block. Five years later, device reprogramming (see Fig. 14.12) revealed the recovery of AV conduction and a dramatic reduction in ventricular pacing. During this period of time the patient was maintained on a stable dose of prednisone and was not on any other immunosuppressant.

Interesting Points

This case illustrates an unusual time course for the recovery of AV conduction in a patient with complete heart block due to cardiac sarcoidosis. This late recovery may have resulted from resolution of inflammation related to granuloma deposition within the interventricular septum with chronic low dose steroid exposure. Importantly, this case emphasizes that patients with complete heart block and cardiac sarcoidosis should be evaluated for recurrent atrioventricular conduction during routine follow-up so that devices can be reprogrammed and forced right-ventricular pacing minimized (Fig. 14.12).

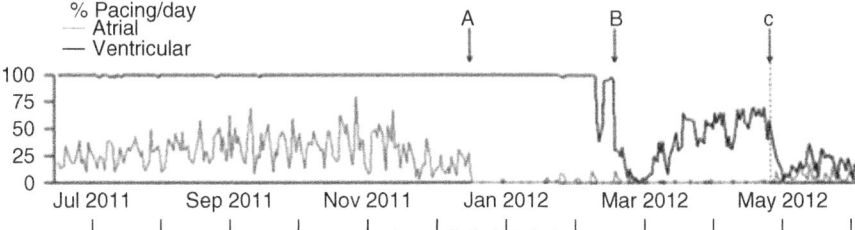

Fig. 14.12 An example of device interrogation data showing recovery of atrioventricular conduction in a patient with cardiac sarcoidosis and a dual-chamber ICD initially placed in the setting of complete atrioventricular block. (*A*) Lower rate reprogrammed to minimize atrial pacing, (*B*) recognition of recovered atrioventricular conduction and longer atrioventricular delay programmed, (*C*) further delay in atrioventricular interval pacing programmed to minimize ventricular pacing

Cardiac Sarcoidosis Clinical Vignette #7

A 61-year old female presented with persistent headache and underwent a computed tomography (CT) of the head and neck for further evaluation. Although there was no obvious source of headache identified, an incidental finding of nodularity in the lung apices was noted. Chest and abdominal CT was performed for further evaluation and revealed significant abdominal lymphadenopathy. Due to a suspicion for lymphoma, a retrocaval biopsy was performed and revealed extensive non-necrotizing granulomatous formation consistent with abdominal sarcoidosis.

Because of complaints of mild palpitations and a concern for concurrent cardiac sarcoidosis (CS), echocardiography was performed. This revealed preserved left ventricular systolic function, left ventricular ejection fraction 61 %, with stage II diastolic dysfunction, and mildly elevated right ventricular systolic pressure (37 mmHg).

A 24 hour Holter monitor was performed and revealed 14,951 premature ventricular complexes (18 % of recorded beats) with 3 and 4 beat runs of non-sustained ventricular tachycardia, heart rate 220 beats per minute, without associated symptoms.

A cardiac magnetic resonance imaging (CMR) study was performed and demonstrated normal left ventricular ejection fraction, LVEF 62 %, with a focus of delayed contrast hyperenhancment in the mid apical lateral wall suggestive of CS (see Fig. 14.13).

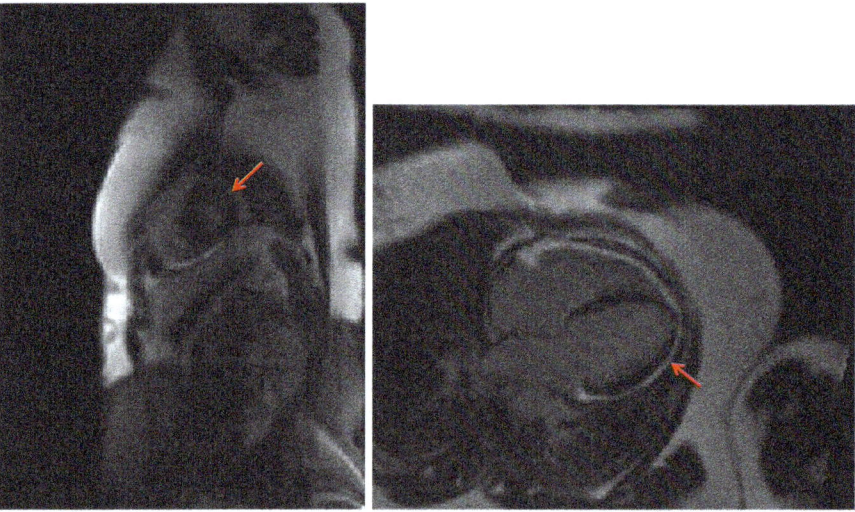

Fig. 14.13 A 61 year old woman with a history of sarcoidosis with mediastinal and abdominal lymphadenopathy. The diagnosis of sarcoidosis was made by retrocaval needle core biopsy with pathology demonstrating non-necrotizing granulomatous inflammation consistent with sarcoidosis. The patient experienced inducible VT/VF and frequent PVCs. Imaging with Cardiac MRI demonstrated mild focal delayed hyperenhancement in the apical lateral wall (*arrows*) suggestive of focal cardiac sarcoidosis. The patient subsequently received an implantable cardioverter defibrillator (ICD)

Subsequently, a right ventricular electrophysiology mapping study and programmed electrical stimulation study were performed which demonstrated inducible polymorphic ventricular tachycardia and fibrillation with low stimulation consistent with CS-associated ventricular dysrhythmia.

A dual chamber internal cardiac defibrillator (ICD) was implanted without complications. Since the ICD implant, the patient has not experienced any ICD discharges or syncope.

Interesting Points

This case highlights the role that CMR can play in the decision to proceed with invasive electrophysiology testing for suspected CS. The combination of palpitations, ventricular tachycardia on non-invasive rhythm monitoring, and a delayed contrast hyperenhancement pattern on CMR that is typical for CS all suggest a high pretest probability of cardiac involvement. However, delayed hyperenhancement that is isolated to more atypical locations for CS such as the mid septal wall can represent other myocardial disease states such as dilated cardiomyopathy and myocarditis. Therefore, caution should be taken to interpret the CMR findings in the context of other clinical signs, symptoms, and findings when determining whether invasive electrophysiologic testing is appropriate.

Cardiac Sarcoidosis Hypertension Clinical Vignette #8

A 45-year old male with a history of transbronchial biopsy-proven Stage IV pulmonary sarcoidosis, tobacco use, and methamphetamine use presented with New York Heart Association (NYHA) functional class III dyspnea. Initial pulmonary function testing demonstrated a severely reduced forced expiratory volume at 1 s (FEV1) of 1.4 L (33 % predicted), a forced vital capacity (FVC) of 2.73 L (50 % predicted), a FEV1/FVC of 51 %, and a diffusion capacity of 40 % predicted, all suggestive of combined obstructive and fibrotic lung disease. Methotrexate and prednisone were initiated for pulmonary sarcoidosis.

Due to a suspicion of sarcoidosis-associated pulmonary hypertension (SAPH), an echocardiogram was performed and revealed severe right ventricular (RV) enlargement, RV pressure overload, RV hypertrophy, and RV systolic dysfunction. Estimated right ventricular systolic pressure (RVSP) was only mildly elevated at 41 mmHg by echocardiogram.

A right heart catheterization demonstrated a mean pulmonary artery pressure of 41 mmHg and a pulmonary capillary wedge pressure of 13 mmHg (see Fig. 14.14).

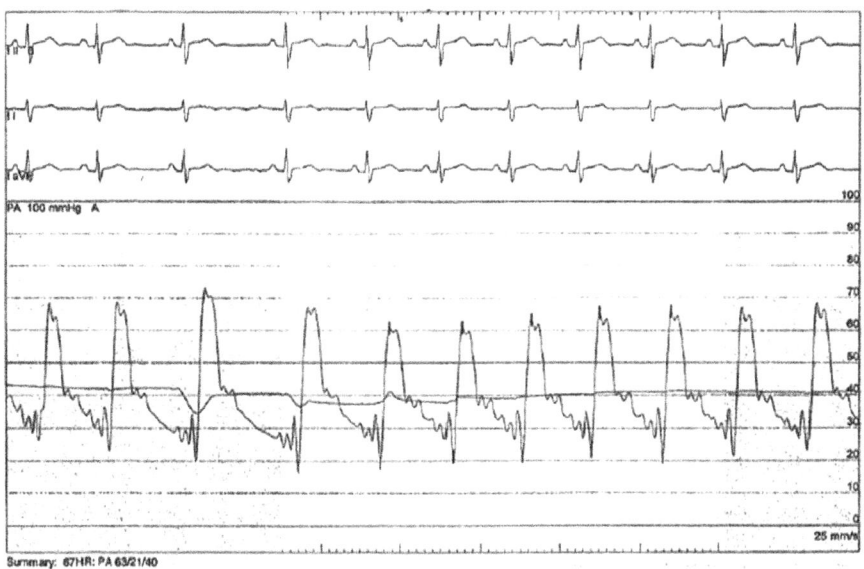

Fig. 14.14 Pulmonary artery pressure waveform from a right heart catheterization in 47 year old man with stage IV pulmonary sarcoidosis and SAPH. The pulmonary artery pressure was 63/21 mmHg (mean 40 mmHg), pulmonary capillary wedge pressure 14 mmHg, and pulmonary vascular resistance of 6 Woods units

The patient was treated with supplemental oxygen, furosemide, spironolactone, and tadalafil. Although he initially improved to NYHA functional class II, his symptoms later progressed.

A repeat right heart catheterization demonstrated essentially no change in hemodynamics: the mean pulmonary artery pressure was 40 mmHg and the pulmonary capillary wedge pressure was 14 mmHg.

The patient could not tolerate combination therapy with ambrisentan or macitentan, due to significant edema, and he was subsequently placed on inhaled iloprost.

Interesting Points

This case highlights the association of SAPH with advanced pulmonary sarcoidosis, the potential for SAPH to overlap with other PH etiologies including chronic obstructive pulmonary disease and methamphetamine use, the limitation of using echocardiogram estimated RVSP to estimate pulmonary artery systolic pressure, and the potential refractory nature of SAPH to conventional PAH therapies.

Cardiac Sarcoidosis Clinical Vignette #9

A 48-year-old female with no prior history of heart disease or systemic cardiac sarcoidosis was referred for cardiac MRI (CMR) to evaluate for potential cause of palpitations and pre-syncope. She also was evaluated with a Holter monitor prior to the CMR study and was found to have one episode of a five beat run of non-sustained ventricular tachycardia.

The CMR study revealed normal left ventricular size and global function (LVEF = 57 %). There were no regional wall motion abnormalities. Late gadolinium enhancement (LGE) images showed a medium amount of subepicardial and mid-wall late gadolinium enhancement involving the basal and inferoseptum at the RV insertion point (Fig. 14.15, red arrow).

There was also a small amount of LGE uptake involving the right ventricular free wall and the basal anteroseptum. The location and multi-focal nature of the LGE findings were strongly suspicious for cardiac sarcoidosis.

Due to suspicion for cardiac sarcoidosis, the patient was referred for PET/CT for further evaluation (see Chap. 6 for explanation of protocol as well as dietary preparation). The whole body and myocardial PET/CT study was performed after an injection of 10 mci of F18-flurodeoxyglucose to assess for metabolism and 22 mci of N13 ammonia to assess resting myocardial perfusion.

The PET/CT images demonstrated a resting perfusion defect involving the basal and mid inferior wall which was matched by increased FDG uptake (red arrow). In addition, there was FDG uptake involving the right ventricular free wall (Fig. 14.16 white arrow), a finding which is associated with an increased risk of adverse events [9]. The whole body FDG images demonstrated mild to moderate focal FDG uptake in both hilar regions and in some mediastinal lymph nodes.

Collectively, the combination of the CMR and PET findings, were diagnostic of cardiac sarcoidosis, and no alternative diagnosis was present to account for these imaging findings. In order to obtain a histological diagnosis, the patient was advised to consider a mediastinal biopsy but declined.

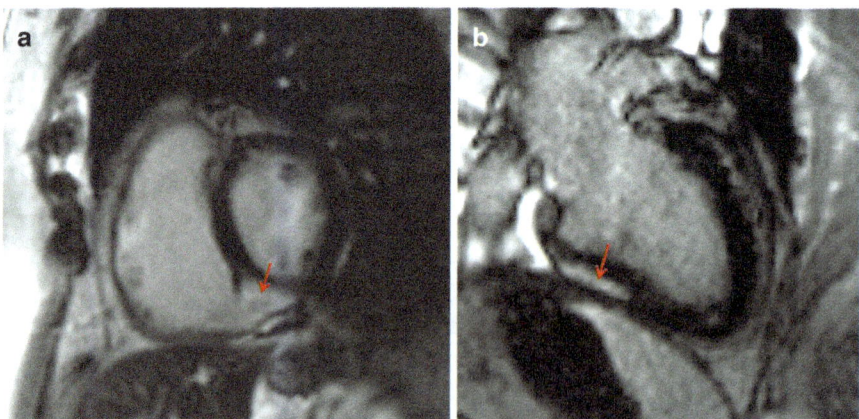

Fig. 14.15 Cardiac MRI late gadolinium enhancement images. (**a**) Basal short axis. (**b**) Two chamber view. See text for explanation of findings

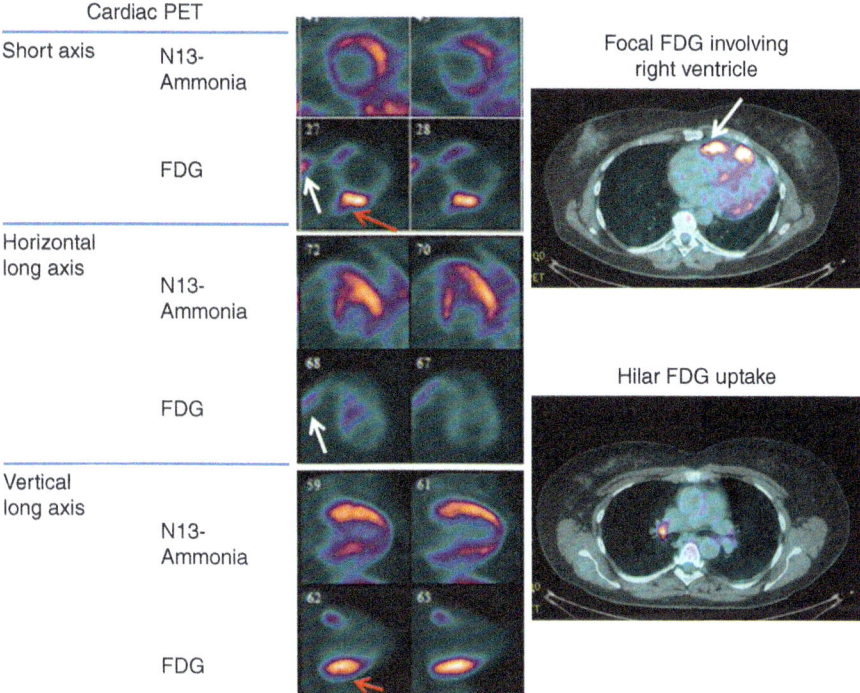

Fig. 14.16 Cardiac PET/CT showing perfusion (N13 ammonia) and metabolism (F18-Flurodeoxyglucose) images. See text for explanation of findings

In this case, given the overwhelming clinical and imaging findings, it was decided to treat the patient for presumed cardiac sarcoidosis despite the absence of a histological diagnosis. Such an approach is often required in taking care of patients with cardiac sarcoidosis, especially given the low yield of endomyocardial biopsy.

Due to the CMR and PET findings the patient was determined to have an increased risk of adverse events and therefore advised to undergo ICD implantation.

She declined due to several concerns, most notably adversity to having a medical device implanted in her body. Several months later, she experienced a syncopal event and upon hospital admission was found to have ventricular tachycardia. She was subsequently treated with ICD implantation as well as started on immunosuppressive therapy.

Interesting Points

As discussed in this guidebook, CMR and PET both visualize different aspects of cardiac sarcoidosis and these tests are often complementary in establishing the diagnosis and prognosis of patients with suspected cardiac involvement. Importantly, abnormalities on these exams, even in the presence of normal left ventricular ejection fraction, is associated with a higher risk of death or ventricular tachycardia.

Cardiac Sarcoidosis Clinical Vignette #10

A 66-year-old white man with a 2 year history of mild non-ischemic cardiomyopathy was admitted for management of recurrent multifocal monomorphic ventricular tachycardia (VT) and worsening systolic function. His initial presentation was of highly symptomatic palpitations related to sustained VT. At the time echocardiography revealed mild LV systolic dysfunction, a coronary angiogram was normal and an ICD was implanted.

Subsequently he failed therapy with sotalol and amiodarone and one attempt at endocardial radiofrequency ablation (RFA) had not reduced his burden of VT. He had no history or clinical evidence of systemic sarcoidosis.

As shown in Fig. 14.17, electrocardiography revealed sinus rhythm with first degree atrio-ventricular (AV) block, left axis deviation, right bundle branch block and bigeminal premature ventricular contractions. Echocardiography (Fig. 14.18) revealed a non-dilated left ventricle, with moderate systolic dysfunction (LVEF 40 %) and mild apical hypokinesis.

Right heart catheterization revealed mildly increased biventricular filling pressures. Endomyocardial biopsy was performed without complication and identified granulomatous myocarditis consistent with sarcoidosis.

FDG-PET (Fig. 14.19) revealed a small size, mild intensity, perfusion defect involving the basal and mid infero-septal walls and FDG revealed diffusely increased myocardial uptake particularly in the basal portion of the heart. Additionally he had FDG avid mediastinal lymph nodes. The SUV max in the LV myocardium 12.3, cerebellar SUV max was 9.3.

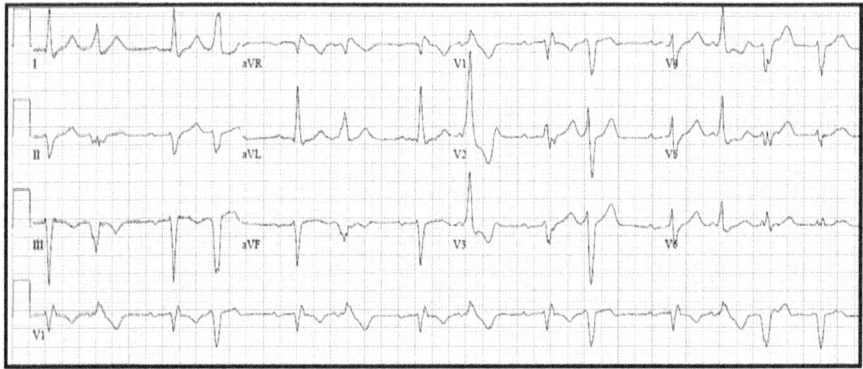

Fig. 14.17 Electrocardiography revealed sinus rhythm with 1st degree atrio-ventricular (*AV*) block, left axis deviation, right bundle branch block and bigeminal premature ventricular contractions

14 Cases in Cardiac Sarcoidosis

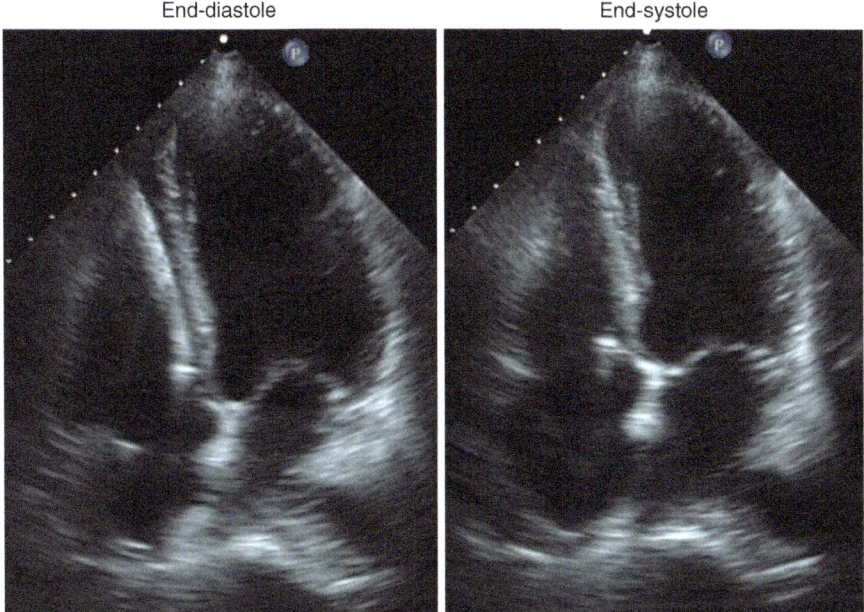

Fig.14.18 Echocardiography revealed a non-dilated left ventricle, with moderate systolic dysfunction (LVEF 40 %) and mild apical hypokinesis

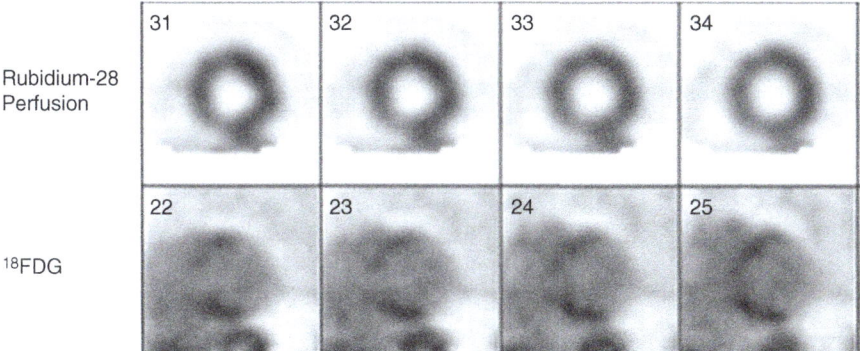

Fig. 14.19 FDG-PET revealed a small size, mild intensity, perfusion defect involving the basal and mid infero-septal walls and FDG revealed diffusely increased myocardial uptake particularly in the basal portion of the heart

Invasive electrophysiology (EP) study identified prolongation of AH (191 ms) and HV (60 ms) intervals. Voltage mapping revealed endocardial and epicardial scars in the posterobasal septum around the tricuspid and mitral annulus. Programmed stimulation induced three different morphologies of VT with left, right and indeterminate bundle morphology. Endocardial and epicaridal radiofrequency energy were applied to multiple areas with substantial abatement, but not elimination of inducible VT. To mitigate future arrhythmia he was treated with metoprolol succinate and mexilitine.

In order to prevent further deterioration in systolic function, conduction disease and recurrent VT, the patient was initiated on prednisone, 0.5 mg/kg, which was gradually tapered to 10 mg daily over 6 months. Prior to initiating prednisone he was tested for latent tuberculosis, bone densitometry was normal and he was taught to check his blood sugar.

Subsequently he developed weight gain, Cushingoid features, proximal muscle weakness and depression. Repeat PET revealed interval decrease in FDG avidity and modest increase in LV systolic function (LVEF 50 %). Low dose methotrexate (15 mg/week) and folic acid (1 mg/day) were substituted for prednisone.

The PR interval remained prolonged and the patient required a second EP study and radiofrequency ablation for management of recurrent VT 6 months after the diagnosis of cardiac sarcoidosis. At that time five different foci were ablated and metoprolol was transitioned to nadolol.

He returned 18 months after diagnosis of CS for routine evaluation. By echocardiography, LVEF remained low normal and there was no suggestion of residual inflammation by FDG PET. He had a modest burden of non-sustained VT on ICD interrogation, but no ICD therapies for VT were required. On this basis methotrexate was discontinued.

Three years after his index presentation, 2 years after prednisone was weaned off and 1 year after methotrexate was discontinued, he has remained clinically stable on mexilitine and nadolol.

He continues to undergo frequent echocardiographic surveillance, but repeat PET was discontinued in lieu of clinical events.

Interesting Points

1. Corticosteroid therapy for cardiac sarcoidosis has been most effective in treating AV block, and less efficacious for VT where scar related reentry is unlikely to be ameliorated by resolution of inflammation [10].
2. Ventricular tachycardia associated with cardiac sarcoidosis is multifocal monomorphic and may require multiple anti-arrhythmic medications and invasive procedures to control [6].
3. Patients should be prepared for the considerable morbidity associated with high dose corticosteroids. Pre-steroid testing should include an assessment for latent tuberculosis infection, osteoporosis and glucose intolerance.

References

1. Sekhri V, et al. Cardiac sarcoidosis: a comprehensive review. Arch Med Sci. 2011;7(4):546–54.
2. Garrett J, O'Neill H, Blake S. Constrictive pericarditis associated with sarcoidosis. Am Heart J. 1984;107:394.
3. Yodogawa K, Seino Y, Ohara T, Takayama H, Katoh T, Mizuno K. Effect of corticosteroid therapy on ventricular arrhythmias in patients with cardiac sarcoidosis. Ann Noninvasive Electrocardiol. 2011;16:140–7.
4. Hamzeh NY, Wamboldt FS, Weinberger HD. Management of cardiac sarcoidosis in the United States: a Delphi study. Chest. 2012;141:154–62.
5. Jefic D, Joel B, Good E, Morady F, Rosman H, Knight B, Bogun F. Role of radiofrequency catheter ablation of ventricular tachycardia in cardiac sarcoidosis: report from a multicenter registry. Heart Rhythm. 2009;6:189–95.
6. Koplan BA, Soejima K, Baughman K, Epstein LM, Stevenson WG. Refractory ventricular tachycardia secondary to cardiac sarcoid: electrophysiologic characteristics, mapping, and ablation. Heart Rhythm. 2006;3:924–9.
7. Stees CS, Khoo MS, Lowery CM, Sauer WH. Ventricular tachycardia storm successfully treated with immunosuppression and catheter ablation in a patient with cardiac sarcoidosis. J Cardiovasc Electrophysiol. 2011;22:210–3.
8. Ohe T. Radiofrequency ablation for ventricular tachycardia in patients with cardiac sarcoidosis: is it worth trying? Heart Rhythm. 2009;6:196–7.
9. Blankstein R, Osborne M, Naya M, et al. Cardiac positron emission tomography enhances prognostic assessments of patients with suspected cardiac sarcoidosis. J Am Coll Cardiol. 2014;63(4):329–336.
10. Sadek MM, Yung D, Birnie DH, Beanlands RS, Nery PB. Corticosteroid therapy for cardiac sarcoidosis: a systematic review. Can J Cardiol. 2013;29:1034–41.

Chapter 15
Patient-Centered Care for Sarcoidosis

Darlene Kim and Howard D. Weinberger

Abstract Caring for patients with sarcoidosis is a challenge. As a relatively rare disorder of unknown etiology, with the potential to affect multiple organ systems in an unpredictable fashion, a patient-centered rather than disease centered approach is very important. Some of the keys to a patient-centered approach include health literacy, patient education, shared decision-making, patient-centered outcomes, and a multidisciplinary team approach which actively involves the patient. These components for a patient-centered approach will be discussed in this chapter.

Patient-Centered Care

Caring for patients with sarcoidosis is a challenge. As a relatively rare disorder of unknown etiology, with the potential to affect multiple organ systems in an unpredictable fashion, a patient-centered approach is very important. Patient-centered care is defined as "care that is respectful of and responsive to individual patient preferences, needs, and values, and ensuring that patient values guide all clinical decisions" [1]. At first glance, the concept seems redundant to the practice of good medicine to warrant deliberate and prescribed reinforcement by the medical community today. However, a twentieth century emphasis on pathophysiology and evidence-based medicine has arguably given rise to medical care that has gradually become "disease-centric." A patient-centered approach is a method of care that places a sharp focus on the patient rather than on the disease, emphasizing effective communication, engagement and empowerment of the patient as an active rather than passive participant in his/her care in addition to empathy, transparency, and a sense of partnership between patient and physician.

D. Kim, MD, FACC (✉) • H.D. Weinberger, MD, FACC, FACP
Division of Cardiology, Department of Medicine, National Jewish Health,
1400 Jackson St., Denver, CO 80206, USA
e-mail: kimd@njhealth.org; weinbergerh@njhealth.org

Health Literacy

Health literacy is key to patient-centered care. Sarcoidosis poses a greater challenge for caregivers to provide information and education to patients compared to a disease process that is better understood. Despite many hypotheses, the cause of sarcoidosis remains unknown to all. Many patients assume that their understanding of sarcoidosis is incomplete rather than realizing that in actuality, our knowledge as an entire medical and scientific community, is incomplete. Effective physician-patient communication that promotes an understanding that we are all "on the same page" in terms of what we know and do not know about sarcoidosis helps to engender a sense of team approach. Communication and understanding here is also critical in terms of discussing current treatment options based on what is known, albeit, incompletely.

Shared Decision-Making

While there is no cure for sarcoidosis today, treatment options exist because we have established that disease propagation is immune-mediated. Health literacy promoting understanding the link between limiting disease progression and the necessity of immunomodulators helps to get the "buy-in" from patients, encouraging patient adherence to a treatment regimen that is born of an understanding of the disease process and treatment. A transparent discussion about the therapeutic benefits as well as potential toxicities of treatment, combined with a thoughtful, individualized weighing of risks and benefits is an example of patient-centered shared decision-making. Similar risk/benefit discussions accounting for radiation exposure and invasiveness of tests and procedures vis-à-vis expected diagnostic and therapeutic benefits should be undertaken at every step.

Patient-Centered Outcomes

Health status encompasses disease activity, functional status, and quality of life. Beyond measurements of disease activity (e.g., pulmonary function tests and echocardiograms), a primary treatment goal in sarcoidosis is the impact of disease status on a patient's symptoms and quality of life. Quality of life is a person's overall satisfaction with issues of importance to him/her, and *distinct* from functional status, which is the ability to perform in physical, social, and mental activities of daily living. Caregivers need to be reminded of quality of life as an important patient-centered endpoint, in addition to disease activity and functional status. The Sarcoidosis Health Questionnaire is a health-related quality of life instrument that was designed specifically for patients with sarcoidosis [2]. It is an assessment that evaluates for daily functioning, physical functioning, and emotional functioning are overlapping parts of a comprehensive evaluation of quality of life. It provides caregivers a way to partly quantify this important end-point, and can open opportunities to discuss areas in which quality of life may be improved, for instance, support groups for patients whose quality of life suffers from a sense of isolation.

Collaborative Care: The Sarcoidosis Team Approach

Because sarcoidosis may affect a variety of organ systems, it is important to involve physicians with experience and interest in sarcoidosis for the care of patients afflicted by this disease. Utilizing a team approach that includes specialists in the areas and organ systems involved will help optimize the patient-centered focus for evaluation, monitoring and management of patients with sarcoidosis, and especially those with cardiac sarcoidosis.

The lead physician should be a sarcoidosis specialist, which will likely be a pulmonologist or perhaps a rheumatologist with interest and experience in identifying, monitoring and treating sarcoidosis. As sarcoidosis primarily affects the lungs, a pulmonologist should be an integral member of the team if a non-pulmonologist is the lead physician. Other specialists with experience and interest in sarcoidosis should be involved based on organ system involvement. As sarcoidosis and some of the treatments for sarcoidosis may often affect the eyes, an ophthalmologist with experience and interest in sarcoidosis should be a part of the team.

For patients with known or suspected cardiac sarcoidosis, a cardiologist with experience and interest in cardiac sarcoidosis is an integral part of the team. This physician will guide diagnostic testing and serial monitoring of cardiac status and will work with the pulmonologist/sarcoidosis specialist in regards to sarcoidosis specific treatment. Standard therapies for cardiovascular disease, including those for heart failure should also be implemented. The sarcoidosis cardiologist will also incorporate cardiology subspecialists such as electrophysiologists and interventional cardiologists as indicated. A cardiac electrophysiologist should be an active participant in the evaluation and management of patients with known or suspected cardiac sarcoidosis, especially in regards to invasive electrophysiology testing for risk stratification, and for arrhythmia and device therapies.

As the evaluation, diagnosis and monitoring of patients with cardiac sarcoidosis involves an array of advanced imaging procedures, a radiologist with expertise in advance imaging as well as sarcoidosis is important. This includes not only standard radiographs and CT scans, but nuclear myocardial perfusion imaging, cardiac magnetic resonance imaging (CMRI) and cardiac 18-FDG PET scanning.

References

1. Institute of Medicine. Crossing the quality chasm: a new health system for the twenty-first century. Washington, DC: The National Academies Press; 2001.
2. Cox CE, et al. The sarcoidosis health questionnaire: a new measure of health-related quality of life. Am J Respir Crit Care Med. 2003;168(3):323–9.

Sarcoidosis Resources for Patients and Caregivers

World Association of Sarcoidosis and other Granulomatous disorders: www.wasog.org	
WASOG journal	Official journal of WASOG "sarcoidosis vasculitis and diffuse lung diseases"
	Includes clinical research, review articles, case reports, and editorials
List of key papers	List of abstracts of selected literature relevant to sarcoidosis
Patient societies	International list of sarcoidosis patient groups
Video	Webinars including key lectures from experts
Newsletter	
Meetings	List of sarcoidosis-related conferences worldwide
Foundation for sarcoidosis research: www.stopsarcoidosis.org	
Patient registry	"Sarcoidosis advanced registry cures," a web-based longitudinal patient registry in progress
Clinical trial connector	List of open trials recruiting patients
Support group directory	Identifies formal support groups worldwide
Patient advocacy and education materials	Informative brochures for patients
Patient conferences and workshops	List of events including awareness walks/runs, fundraisers, conferences
Physicians' treatment protocol	Handy treatment guidelines reference document and mobile app

Index

A
A Case Control Etiologic Sarcoidosis Study (ACCESS study), 5–6
Acute management, of cardiac sarcoidosis
   cardiac manifestations in patients with
      hitherto unknown systemic sarcoidosis, 95
      isolated cardiac sarcoidosis, 96–97
      known systemic sarcoidosis, 94–95
   corticosteroids, 97
      atrioventricular block, 98
      testing and management for, 99
      ventricular tachycardia, 98–99
      worsening systolic function, 99–100
   diagnostic criteria, 94, 95
   immunosuppressive agents, 98
   sarcoidosis evaluation, 97
   steroid sparing agents, 97
Ambulatory electrocardiographic monitoring, 19–20
American College of Cardiology Foundation (ACCF), 75–76
American Heart Association (AHA), 75–76
Angiotensin-converting enzyme (ACE) genes, 6
Antitumor necrosis factor-alpha (Anti-TNF-α), 106–107
Arrhythmias management
   atrial arrhythmias, 85–87
   conduction system disease
      atrioventricular block, 84–85
      bundle branch block, 82
      catheter ablation of, 89
      electrocardiographic progression of, 82–84
      sinus node dysfunction, 85, 86
   ventricular arrhythmias
      anti-arrhythmic drugs, 88–89
      corticosteroids, 88–89
      granuloma infiltration, 88
      pleomorphic ventricular tachycardia, 88
      worsening of, 145
Atrial arrhythmias
   anti-arrhythmic therapy, 87
   catheter ablation of, 87
   mechanism of, 86–87
   prevalence of, 85, 87
Atrioventricular block, 84–85, 98
Atrioventricular (AV) conduction, recovery of, 149
Automated implantable cardioverter defibrillator (AICD), 145
Azathioprine, 107, 109

B
Bundle branch block, 82

C
Cardiac catheterization, 73–74
Cardiac magnetic resonance imaging (CMR), 154, 155
   delayed contrast hyperenhancement, 142
   with delayed gadolinium, 76
   extracardiac findings, 32
   features and disease pattern
      acute inflammation, 29
      post-inflammatory scarring, 29, 30
      pulmonary hypertension, 31
      wall motion abnormality, 31

Cardiac magnetic resonance
    imaging (CMR) (cont.)
  first imaging strategy, 60–63
  left ventricular ejection fraction, 150–151
  limitations for, 32, 33
  myocardial DHE diagnosis, 31
  post-processing, 28
  prognostic value of, 59–60, 64
  protocol/sequences, 27–28
  role of, 25–26
  SCD risk stratification, 116
  steroid therapy, 67
  techniques, 26–28
  T2 weighted imaging, 25
Cardiac PET/CT, 154, 155
  hypermetabolic activity, 33–34
  pre-exam patient instructions, 32–33
Cardiac sarcoidosis, 3
  clinical presentations, 11–13
  complete heart block, 12
  valvular dysfunction, 12–13
Collaborative care, 163
Complete atrioventricular block (CAVB), 84–85
Complete heart block
  clinical presentation, 11, 12
  electrocardiogram, 16, 136
Conduction system disease
  atrioventricular block, 84–85
  bundle branch block, 82
  catheter ablation of, 89
  electrocardiographic progression of, 82–84
  sinus node dysfunction, 85, 86
Corticosteroids, 97
  atrioventricular block, 98
  granulomas, 138
  left ventricular function, 105
  testing and management for, 99
  for ventricular arrhythmias, 88, 89
  ventricular tachycardia, 98–99
  worsening systolic function, 99–100

D
Delayed hyperenhancement (DHE) imaging, 27
Delphi study, 107, 108

E
Electroanatomical mapping (EAM), 77–78
Electroanatomical voltage map, 147
Electrocardiography (ECG), 16–19
  complete heart block, 136
  of conduction system disease, 82–84

  first degree AV block, 140, 156
  Mobitz type 2 second-degree
    AV block, 138, 139
  multimodality imaging, 55–56
  non-dilated left ventricle, 156, 157
  patients with sinus node
    dysfunction, 85, 86
  sarcoidosis-associated pulmonary
    hypertension, 128, 129
Electrophysiology (EP) study
  AH and HV prolongation, 158
  patients with extra-cardiac sarcoidosis, 74
Endomyocardial biopsy, 20, 74, 137
  AHA/ACCF/ESC joint statement, 75–76
  clinical scenarios, 76
  delayed gadolinium enhancement, 138
  electroanatomical mapping-guided
    biopsy, 77–78
  imaging-guided biopsies, 76–77
  major and minor complications, 75
European Society of Cardiology
    (ESC), 75–76

F
^{18}F-fluoro-2-deoxyglucose positron emission
    tomography (^{18}F-FDG PET)
  active inflammation/damage., 76
  patchy inflammation, 143
  SCD risk stratification, 116
F18-Flurodeoxyglucose (F18-FDG), 41
First-degree atrio-ventricular (AV) block, 140
18-flouro-deoxuyglucose positron emission
    tomography (FDG-PET), 156–157
  image interpretation, 43–46
  with MPI
    acquisition protocol for, 56–57
    focal areas of, 58
    immunosuppression therapy, 67
    interpretation of, 57
    quantitative interpretation of, 59
  patient preparation, 41–42
  protocol, 42–43
  quantifying methods, 69
  therapy response, 45–47

G
Gadolinium, 59
Gallium-67 imaging, 40
Giant cell myocarditis (GCM), 97
Granulomas
  corticosteroids, 138
  endomyocardial biopsy, 138
  in SAPH, 126

Index

H
Health literacy, 161–162
Holter monitoring, 19, 54, 138, 150
Hypertension, 136–137

I
ICD. *See* Implantable cardiac defibrillator (ICD)
Immunosuppressive (IS) therapy
   Delphi study, 107
   electrocardiographic changes, 104–105
   indication of, 104
   left ventricular function, 105
   on survival, 105–106
   therapy duration, 106–107
Implantable cardiac defibrillator (ICD)
   incidence, 119
   indications for, 117
   nested case-control study, 118
   observational studies, 118
   recommendations, 114
   sensed R-waves, 120
   sudden cardiac death, 113
   ventricular arrhythmias, 88
International Society of Heart Lung Transplant, 131
Iodine-123-labeled 15-(p-iodophenyl)-3R, S-methylpentadecanoic acid (BMIPP), 47

J
Japanese Ministry of Health and Welfare (JMHW) criteria, 16, 94, 104

L
Late gadolinium enhancement (LGE), 59
Leflunomide, 109
Left ventricular (LV) function, 105
Left ventricular systolic function (LVEF), 115–116

M
Methotrexate, 106
Mobitz type 2 second-degree AV block, 138, 139
MPI. *See* Myocardial perfusion imaging (MPI)
Multimodality imaging
   abnormal screening studies, 54
   cardiac MRI, 59–60
   CMR first strategy, 60–63
   echocardiography, 55–56
   fundamental data publication, 68–69
   imaging role in, 52
   non-invasive imaging, 52
   nuclear imaging techniques, 56–59
   patient indication, 53
   patients with known cardiac sarcoidosis, 66
   prognostic value, 63–66
   systemic sarcoidosis incidence, 53
   therapy response, 66–68
Mycophenolate mofetil, 107, 109
Myocardial perfusion imaging (MPI)
   FDG PET with
      acquisition protocol for, 56–57
      focal areas of, 58
      immunosuppression therapy, 67
      interpretation of, 57
      quantitative interpretation of, 59
   use of, 40–41

N
N-13 ammonia, 40, 44
New York Heart Association (NYHA), 106
Non-sustained ventricular tachycardia (NSVT), 138, 146
Nuclear imaging
   FDG PET imaging (*see* 18-flouro-deoxuyglucose positron emission tomography (FDG-PET))
   F18-FDG, 41
   Gallium-67, 40
   rest MPI, 40–41

P
PAH. *See* Pulmonary arterial hypertension (PAH)
Patient-centered care
   collaborative care, 163
   definition, 161
   health literacy, 161–162
   outcomes, 162
   shared decision-making, 162
Positron emission tomography (PET)
   prognostic value of, 64–65
   rest MPI, 40
   SCD risk stratification, 116, 117
Prednisone, 107
Propionibacterium, 8
Prostacyclin, 131
Pulmonary arterial hypertension (PAH), 125
Pulmonary artery pressure waveform, 131
Pulmonary hypertension (PH), 125
Pulmonary vasodilators, 130–131

Q
Quality of life, 162

R
Right ventricular systolic function (RVEF), 115–116
Right ventricular systolic pressure (RVSP), 127
Rubidium-82, 40

S
SAECG. *See* Signal-averaged ECG (SAECG)
SAPH. *See* Sarcoidosis-associated pulmonary hypertension (SAPH)
Sarcoidosis
  clinical manifestations, 8
  description, 1
  differential diagnosis of, 7
  epidemiology, 1–3
  etiologies of, 7
  pathophysiology
    familial clusters of, 5–6
    T-cell and T-cell receptor pathology, 6
    vitamin D receptor polymorphisms, 6
Sarcoidosis-associated pulmonary hypertension (SAPH), 125
  diagnosis, 129
  electrocardiography, 128, 129
  epidemiology, 126
  evaluation, 127–129
  pathophysiology, 126–127
  prognosis, 132
  prostacyclin, 131
  pulmonary artery pressure, 152–153
  treatment, 129–132
  WHO classification system, 126
Sarcoidosis Health Questionnaire, 162
SCD. *See* Sudden cardiac death (SCD)
Screening for cardiac sarcoidosis
  ambulatory electrocardiographic monitoring, 19–20
  echocardiography, 18–19
  electrocardiography, 16–17
  endomyocardial biopsy, 20
  positive imaging result, 22
  SAECG, 17–18
  scoring system, 21
Shared decision-making, 162
Signal-averaged ECG (SAECG), 17–18, 84
Single-photon emission computed tomography (SPECT) imaging, 34–36
  Gallium-67, 40
  rest MPI, 40
Sinus node dysfunction, 85
Standard Uptake Values (SUV), 67–68
Steroid sparing agents, 97, 98, 109
ST-T wave abnormalities, 140, 141
Sudden cardiac death (SCD), 113
  implantable cardiac defibrillator, 113
  incidence, 119
  indications for, 117
  nested case-control study, 118
  observational studies, 118
  recommendations, 114
  sensed R-waves, 120
  risk stratification, 114–117
    with cardiac imaging, 116
    electrophysiologic testing, 117
    LV/RV systolic function, 115–116
Supraventricular arrhythmias, 85–86

T
Team approach, sarcoidosis, 163
Technetium-99m, 40
Technetium (99mTc) sestamibi, 34–36

V
Ventricular arrhythmias
  anti-arrhythmic drugs, 88–89
  corticosteroids, 88–89
  granuloma infiltration, 88
  pleomorphic ventricular tachycardia, 88
Ventricular tachycardia, 98–99
Vitamin D receptor polymorphisms, 6

The manufacturer's authorised representative in the EU is Springer Nature Customer Service Centre GmbH, Europaplatz 3, 69115 Heidelberg, Germany. If you have any concerns regarding our products, please contact ProductSafety@springernature.com

Printed and bound by CPI Group (UK) Ltd, Croydon, CR0 4YY

23/03/2026

02076369-0010